INFECTIOUS PROCESS AND SEPSIS

Edited by **Vincenzo Neri**

Infectious Process and Sepsis
http://dx.doi.org/10.5772/intechopen.77750
Edited by Vincenzo Neri

Contributors

Giorgio Berlot, Natalia Beloborodova, Ekaterina Chernevskaya, Dablulal Gupta, D.N. Rao, Sanjeev Bhoi, Tejprakash Sinha, Bashir A. Bashir, Reinhold P. Linke, Vincenzo Neri, Silvia Passero

First published in London, United Kingdom, 2020 by IntechOpen
IntechOpen is the global imprint of INTECHOPEN LIMITED, registered in England and Wales, registration number: 11086078, 7th floor, 10 Lower Thames Street, London,
EC3R 6AF, United Kingdom
Printed in Croatia

British Library Cataloguing-in-Publication Data
A catalogue record for this book is available from the British Library

Additional hard and PDF copies can be obtained from orders@intechopen.com

Infectious Process and Sepsis, Edited by Vincenzo Neri
p. cm.
Print ISBN 978-1-83880-393-3
Online ISBN 978-1-83880-394-0
eBook (PDF) ISBN 978-1-83962-983-9

For EU product safety concerns:
IN TECH d.o.o., Prolaz Marije Krucifikse Kozulić 3, 51000 Rijeka, Croatia,
info@intechopen.com or visit our website at intechopen.com.

Meet the editor

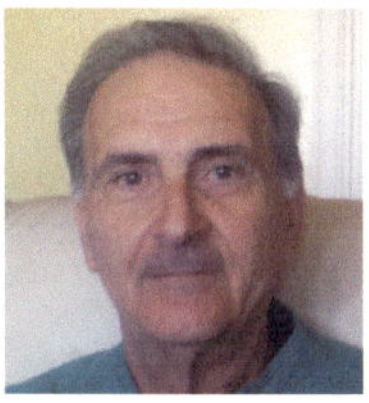

Vincenzo Neri is a former professor (retired) of General Surgery at the Department of Medical and Surgical Sciences (from 2002), Director of Division of General Surgery (from 1997), Director of Residency School of General Surgery (from 2008), Director of Department of Surgical Sciences (2002–2008), and President of Course of Degree of Medicine and Surgery (1996–2002) at University of Foggia, Italy. He was previously Assistant Professor (1974–1982) and Associate Professor (1982–2001) at the School of Medicine and Surgery, University of Bari, Italy. He graduated in Medicine and Surgery (1970) and completed postgraduate training in General Surgery (1975) and Emergency Surgery (1979) at University of Bari, Italy. He received a diploma of "Maitrise Universitaire en Pedagogie des Sciences de la Santè" from the University Paris-Nord Bobigny (1995). His main research interest is hepatobiliarypancreatic surgery, specifically the management of acute pancreatitis and treatment of pancreatic and liver tumors. He has published research papers, reviews, congress proceedings, and book chapters. He attended, in the period 1991–2016, for short periods every year, the Hepatobiliarypancreatic Surgery Service of Beaujon Hospital, Universitè de Paris, Clichy. He developed a seminar on "Cystic Tumours of the Pancreas" for the Erasmus Program at Ghent University, Belgium, in 2010–2011. He is a member of Societa' Italiana di Chirurgia (SIC), International Hepatopancreatobiliary Association (IHPBA), European Association for the Study of Liver (EASL), New European Surgical Academy (NESA), Society of Laparoscopic & Robotic Surgeons (SLS).

Contents

Preface

Sepsis is as a complex body response to infectious agents (bacteria, virus, fungi, multicellular parasites, etc.). The human species, as all mammals, has three defense mechanisms against pathogens: anatomical barriers, nonspecific immunity, and specific immunity. The anatomical barriers are the skin; the mucous surface, such as conjunctiva and the oral cavity with the protection of lysozyme; the mucous layer of the respiratory tract, secreted by muciparous cells, and removed by eyelashes; and the acidic environment in the stomach, vagina, and on the skin. The first step of the organism reaction is tissue response to the damage caused by foreign viable agents that have passed the anatomical barriers, the body's first defense, or by pathological action of endogenous agents, present as commensals in various organs. This response is called inflammation and its purpose is to bring in the damaged site cells and serum molecules. The inflammation develops through the following phases: increment of hematic perfusion in the site, increase of capillary permeability, and cellular migration from blood vessels to tissues. The inflammation is a local reaction and the results are positive, mostly because its action is confined in a site. The next phase of inflammation, after increase of perfusion, is the nonspecific cellular response. The macrophages and neutrophils are the main cells that perform the action of phagocytosis of pathogens. Viral infections cause, by various cellular types, the secretion of an antiviral substance called interferon that prevents viral multiplication in the cells. Many pathogens induce the multifactorial tissue response of acute inflammation; in fact, if surface protection mechanisms and nonspecific cellular mechanisms fail to prevent invasion of pathogenic microorganisms, specific defined immune responses go into action. Many pathogens can activate specific immune responses. The activation of the immune system leads the recognition of particular characteristics of specific pathogens that are specific surface macromolecules, called antigens. Therefore the antigens produce responses, antibodies, intended to destroy them and the pathogen. This last phase of the organism's response takes place in the systemic dimension. The systemic involvement of specific immune responses can evolve in the onset of systemic inflammatory response and sepsis, which is conditioned in its severity by the response of the organism, amplified by the cascade of inflammation mediators. In this way, severe sepsis and septic shock can develop.

The introductory chapter "Surgical Infections" summarizes the pathogenesis, defense mechanisms, and clinical problems of autonomous infectious pathologies of single organs treated with surgical procedures, wound infections, and surgical site infections. The chapter "Immunodepression in Sepsis" focuses on the down-regulation of the innate and adaptive immune capabilities caused by anti-inflammatory substances. It emphasizes the control of the immune system and the perspectives of therapeutic strategies. The chapter "Microbiota-Oriented Diagnostics and Therapy in Sepsis: Utopia or Necessity" regards the disruption of microbiota as an indicator of the role they play in sepsis. The changes of the gut microbiota and the characteristics of interactions in the septic microbiome can allow advances in diagnosis and therapy of sepsis. The chapter "Cytokine Gene Polymorphism and Sepsis" discusses the importance of cytokines for host immune response. The study suggests that variations in the promoter and structural regions of cytokine genes are involved in the inflammatory responses and in inter-individual differences in sepsis severity. The chapter "Hemostatic Aspects of Sepsis" analyzes the changes of the hemostatic system under septic conditions, such as coagulopathy with disseminated intravascular coagulation and increase of developing organ dysfunction, morbidity, and mortality. The final chapter, "The Invariant Peptide Clusters of Serum Amyloid A Are Humoral Checkpoints for Vital Innate Functions as Probed by Monoclonal Antibodies, Including in Sepsis: Induction by Febrile Temperatures and Path of Discoveries," subdivides the argument in sections and subsections and clarifies the complex topic of the role of serum amyloid A in the acute phase of sepsis.

Prof. Vincenzo Neri
University of Foggia, Italy

Chapter 1

Introductory Chapter: Surgical Infections

Vincenzo Neri

Additional information is available at the end of the chapter

http://dx.doi.org/10.5772/intechopen.92259

1. Introduction

Surgical infections are infectious diseases that can be treated with surgical procedures or occur in the surgical site. Synthetically, these are a localized, closed infectious disease. In the first group, the autonomous infectious pathologies of single organs or closed sites, as abscesses, appendicitis, cholecystitis, colonic diverticulitis, etc., are included. However, in the other group, there are the surgical site infections, surgical wound infections, etc. It is important to remind that the post-surgical infections can develop as local disease or as general disease with startup of systemic inflammatory response syndrome (SIRS) and then sepsis, severe sepsis, and septic shock. The surgical site and wound infections can come from the external environment or from an endogenous contamination. The infections from external environment, hospital ward, operating room, and surgical equipment, are controlled and resolved by sterilization procedures. Very crucial is the role of perioperative nurses, which should control and save the sterile techniques, detect the occurred breaks, and communicate actively to all team members. Less easily the contaminations from endogenous infective agents, pathologic aerobes and anaerobes, that are present, as commensals, in the digestive, biliary and urinary tract, airways, etc., can be controlled. In the perspective of infective risk, surgical procedures have been subdivided into four types. This classification enables proper risk stratification of occurrence of infective complications [1]. Obviously, this risk is not only connected with the environmental or endogenous sources of contamination involved during surgical procedures, but is conditioned by the general conditions of patients, characteristics of occurred intraoperative contamination, etc. [2]. The surgical procedures are classified as following: class I clean intervention—during these procedures, there is no opening of the lumen of intestinal, urinary, respiratory, genital tract; also there is no treatment for inflamed tissues or septic outbreaks. Among these interventions, there are abdominal parietal hernias, thyroid and breast surgery, exploratory abdominal surgery, etc. Class II clean-contaminated intervention—in this class, interventions during which the opening of digestive, urinary, and respiratory tract is scheduled, with checked normal situation and without uncommon contamination are collected. We can list in this the following: group biliary tract, urinary tract, gynecological surgery, appendectomy, etc. Class III contaminated intervention—this section encompasses the procedures with prolonged opening of digestive, biliary, and urinary tract, especially with major leak of intestinal or biliary content. Also there is the presence and treatment of inflamed sites. Usually large bowel surgery should be inserted in this class. Class IV dirty-infected intervention—this includes all surgical procedures for acute peritonitis, with septic collections, pus, and fecal contamination: ultimately all the pathologies with severe septic contamination to be treated by surgery [3].

2. Pathogenesis

In the clinical scenario of the surgical infections, some factors are in evidence: infectious agents, the patient's immune defenses, and finally, but most important, the physiopathological characteristics of the site of infections, for example, the type of site perfusion. The infections agents are bacteria, virus, fungi, etc. Their involvement can develop as contamination from outside the body or with the assumption of active pathogenetic function of endogenous infective agents and development of disease. The list of possible infectious agents is very long and varied. Aerobic bacteria are steadily on the skin. *Staphylococcus aureus* is always present in wounds infections. *Streptococcus* penetrates usually in the skin's lesions, fractures, and interests connective tissue [4], following which the bacteria invasion of the connective tissue develops a complex vascular, lymphatic, and local tissue reaction which is defined as inflammation. This is a basic reaction to injury is caused by a foreign and deleterious agent and is intended to locate and destroy it. When inflammation is caused by viable agent (bacteria, virus, etc.), it may be considered as the physical basis of infectious process. The morphological picture of inflammation can suggest that inflammation is a relatively static phenomenon. The viable agents in contact with the tissue will cause an inflammatory reaction of various degree of severity, from hyperemia to serious suppurative process. The first step of inflammation process is the alteration of local fluid exchange by an increase of capillary permeability. There is an immunological action of inflammation process, with the purpose to limit the bacteria, firstly by the initial increase of capillary permeability: with the increased passage of plasma protein, there is the accumulation of fibrinogen in the site of lesion, the formation of fibrous network, and occlusion of draining lymphatics by trombi. In this way, the site of inflammation is confined and limited. The celerity and effectiveness of the process of boundary are very important in the control of diffusion of the pathological microorganisms [5]. The staphylococcus is a very damaging agent but in turn causes rapid local fixation and poor dissemination. On the contrary the hemolytic *Streptococcus*, with a local bland action, is consequently more invasive. The role of inflammation in immunity is a control in bacterial invasiveness. Anaerobic microorganisms are more frequently identified in surgical infections. The important pathologic anaerobes with clinical role are *Clostridium*, *Bacteroides*, *Fusobacterium*, *Peptostreptococcus*. All these bacteria are commensals and therefore the origin of anaerobic infections is endogenous; especially in the colon, the anaerobic flora is largely prevalent. We have to add, for its great diffusion, also the *Escherichia coli*, which is anaerobic/aerobic. In fact, *Escherichia coli*, an enteric microorganism, and other enterococci are often detected together with anaerobes in the surgical infections. The most frequent anaerobic surgical infections are the complications of abdominal surgery, as wound infections after large bowel and gynecological surgery, and intra-abdominal septic collections especially caused by anastomotic leakage. The characteristics of anaerobic infections are the presence of putrid exudate, feculent odor, and gas production [6]. In the immunosuppressed patients, the role of opportunistic bacteria Pseudomonas and Serratia is preeminent, which are external surface contaminants, but usually nonpathogenic. A particular problem is the possible peripheral dissemination of bacteria in case of contaminated wounds. *Streptococcus* bacteria release around the infected site speedily. On the contrary, *Escherichia coli* and *Staphylococcus* are more slower. In this septic scenario, the surgical action of the debridement in the infected wounds is in evidence. With debridement, all devitalized tissues from the site are removed. This action is important because the phagocytic activity of neutrophils in the site of inflammation is more efficacious in reducing the bacteria dissemination if the devitalized tissues have been removed [7]. Also fungi, yeasts, and parasites (*Echinococcus, Amoeba*) can cause infestations; sometime, these develop in the septic collections, abscesses, which require the surgical procedures. The tuberculous infections, usually treated with pharmacological therapy, may be treated by surgery in cases of drug-resistant forms, sequelae of pulmonary tuberculosis, pulmonary aspergilloma, nonfunctioning tuberculous kidney, etc.

3. Host's defense mechanisms

The autonomous infectious diseases of single organs and the surgical site infections, surgical wound infections, in each class of risk, are affected in their clinical evolution by some predisposing conditions. Defective or missing control of external contaminations and imperfect check of intraoperative contaminations have been previously considered. In this scenario, the state and the condition of host's defense mechanisms are certainly crucial. The control of environmental source of contamination can be obtained by strict observance of sterilization procedures of ward, operating room, surgical equipment and devices, etc. To avoid or minimize the risk of intraoperative contaminations, it is decisive to follow the specified well-known procedures for each surgical intervention. More complex is the evaluation of host's defense mechanisms. The first obstacle to infections is the integrity of anatomical barriers: the skin and mucous membranes. Beside anatomical barriers, the immunity system is at the heart of defense mechanisms. Usually, the immunity in the scientific treaties is subdivided into nonspecific and specific immunity. The nonspecific immunity is based on the phagocytic activity of reticuloendothelial system which encompasses distributed phagocytes in the various organs: circulating monocytes and macrophages, polymorphonuclear granulocytes, neutrophils, connective tissue and mucosa mast cells, Kupffer cells in the liver, etc. The phagocytes incorporate pathogenic microorganisms, foreign materials, and cellular debris and destroy them. The macrophages also transport the antigen to the lymph nodes where this stimulates the lymphocytes. The antibodies, secreted by B lymphocytes and bound to particles, favor the recognition of the latter by phagocytes. These accessory cells play a predominant role in killing parasites and in controlling inflammatory processes. The mast cells and basophils contain various molecules which are mediators of inflammation. Consequently, they are very important in the correlations between immune responses and inflammatory reactions [8]. The specific immunity synthetically develops through some phases: the exposition to an antigen (foreign body with antigenic capacity, such as bacteria, viruses, etc.) and afterward recognition and processing of antigen by macrophages, entered into action of T and B lymphocytes, and subsequently, synthesis of specific antibody. The impairment, also in a specific phase, of this multifactorial process causes the global alteration of the immunity functions, the immunodeficiency, which can concur in increased severity of surgical infections. The lymphocytes play a central role in the control of immune response. They specifically recognize antigens distinguishing them from the body's own components. There are two lines of lymphocytes: B cells that produce antibodies and T cells that have various functions—assist B cells in the production of antibodies, recognize and destroy infected virus cells, activate phagocytes for the destruction of pathogens, and check the level and quality of the immune response [9]. Synthetically the inflammation is the response of a tissue to a damage and is meant to bring serum molecules and immune system cells to the damaged site. The flogosis encompasses local increase in blood perfusion and vasodilation, increased capillary permeability, and cells migration from blood vessels to tissues. In this process, some phases develop, as vasodilation, tissue oozing, exudation, marginalization, diapedesis, and chemotaxis; the latter can be defined as movement of cells in response to chemoattractive molecules. These acute phase proteins are various: PCR, interferons, interleukin, etc. Then, phagocytosis follows: the cells incorporate particles and microorganisms. The phases of phagocytosis are the following: adhesion to phagocytes of particles through nonspecific receptors or through opsonization by antibodies and/or complement and adhesion by receptors for Fc, C3b, and C3bi; then, phagosome formation, fusion of lysosome (damage and digestion), and release of microbial products [10].

4. Systemic inflammatory response syndrome: clinical evolution of sepsis

Sepsis is a clinical syndrome initiated by immune system and coagulation, caused by the presence of bacterial or viral infection. Severe sepsis can be defined as organ dysfunction or tissue hypoperfusion due to sepsis, requiring intensive therapy. Septic shock is a severe condition characterized by hemodynamic instability, hypotension, and despite the adequate infusion of fluids, as evolution of organs dysfunction and sepsis. Most frequent causes of severe sepsis are pulmonary infections, intestinal perforations, and urinary and skin infections. Severe sepsis requires the diagnostic quick recognition and starting treatment in the early stages. It can be briefly stated that sepsis and its worsening evolutions are the result of systemic inflammatory response, resulting from an infection (systemic inflammatory response syndrome, SIRS). The diagnosis of sepsis requires at least two of the following signs: body temperature more than 38°C or less than 36°C, heart rate more than 90 bm, breath frequency more than 20 bm, and white blood cells more than 12,000 or less than 4000. Keep in mind that SIRS can be triggered not only by infection but also by numerous other factors as trauma, burns, pancreatitis, etc. However, not all infections cause sepsis, which is conditioned by the body's inflammatory response. In fact there is different degree of inflammatory response to infection and therefore it is necessary to distinguish the infection accompanied by physiological response of the organism, such as fever for small localized infections, from infections accompanied by an abnormal and exaggerated, therefore negative, inflammatory systemic response (SIRS), with start of organ dysfunction [11]. The sequential-sepsis-related organ failure assessment (SOFA) score allows to quantitatively evaluate organ damage. The assessment of the progressive alterations of the clinical function indexes of six organ system allows to evaluate, in the evolution of the sepsis, four severity classes. The score SOFA is based on the assessment of the function of each organ system by means of the appropriate measuring medium: Respiratory, PaO_2/FiO_2, mmHg-coagulation, platelets, $\times$10,000/mm—liver, bilirubin, mg/dL—cardiovascular, mean arterial pressure (MAP) + amine support—central nervous system, Glasgow Coma Scale—renal, creatinine, mg/dL + urine output, mL/d. A score from 0 (normal condition) to 4 for increasing severity is assigned to each of the indices that report the functional condition of the six organ system. The baseline score is 0; the score 2 indicates already organ dysfunction, with 10% mortality; higher scores indicate serious functional impairment. In clinical practice, the quickSOFA has been proposed; it allows to more easily identify the patients at risk of developing septic status. The quickSOFA regards only three parameters of immediate clinical finding: Tachypnea—breath frequency more than 22 bm arterial pressure—less than 100 mmHg Glasgow Coma Scale—less than 15 (it ranges from 3 to 15; higher score indicates better neuro condition) [12]. It is necessary to briefly clarify the mechanism and timing of systemic inflammatory syndrome which from a simple localized infection can lead to the septic state. In this process, bacteria and endotoxins play the role of the triggers of the onset of systemic inflammation and sepsis, which is conditioned by the response of organism, as the trigger causes for the evolution and severity of subsequent events [13]. The cascade of inflammation mediators is activated and the inflammatory response is amplified. The systemic inflammation evolves in three steps. The first step is the trigger of inflammation, characterized by the intracellular activation of trypsinogen to trypsin, by zymogen-lysosomal granule. In the second step, the systemic inflammatory response develops; some phenomena follow: activated digestive enzymes in the blood circulation are present, chemokines in the secretory vesicles released by damaged or infected cells chemoattract inflammatory cells, and neutrophils-macrophages release cytokines. Therefore they develop: local inflammatory response with increased vascular permeability, hemorrhage, necrosis and systemic inflammatory response with the development of SIRS, MODS, toxic phase. Finally in the third step, there is the systemic infections response with the compensatory anti-inflammatory response syndrome (CARS), which is a complex and not a well-defined plan of immunologic responses to severe sepsis [13]. High mortality of septic shock is linked to multi-organ dysfunction, lung, kidney, liver, digestive system, heart, brain, and vascular system. The beginning of multi-organ dysfunction is very variable and unpredictable. In fact, it can be precipitated or slow and sneaky. The number of organs involved in the dysfunctional process and the time of the dysfunction condition the prognosis that progressively worsens with the increase of involved organs: if the involved organs are two, the mortality reaches 32%; it rises to 67% for three organs and finally to 90% in case of four or more organs. The mortality index rises significantly due to prolongation of dysfunction over 24–48 h. The evolution of systemic inflammatory syndrome, which underlies the multiple organ dysfunction syndrome (MODS) is favored by impaired general conditions of patients: old age, immune impairment, and active comorbidities as cardiovascular, renal, hepatic, metabolic pathologies [11].

Author details

Vincenzo Neri

Address all correspondence to: vincenzo.neri@unifg.it

University of Foggia, Italy

References

[1] Devaney L, Rowell K. Improving surgical wound classification—Why it matters. AORN Journal. 2004;**80**:208-223

[2] Anaya DA, Dellinger RP. Challenges in the prevention of the surgical site infections. Infections in Medicine. 2006;**23**:120-126

[3] Onyekwelu I, Yakkanti R, Protzer L, et al. Surgical wound classification and surgical site infections in the orthopaedic patient. JAAOS Global Research & Reviews. 2017;**1**:e022

[4] Giacometti A, Cirioni O, Schimizzi AM, et al. Epidemiology and microbiology of surgical wound infections. Journal of Clinical Microbiology. 2000;**38**:918-922

[5] Bowler PG, Duerden BI, Armstrong DG, et al. Wound microbiology and associated approaches to wound management. Clinical Microbiology Reviews. 2001;**14**:244-269

[6] Cooper RA. Surgical site infections: Epidemiology and microbiological aspects in traoma and orthopaedic surgery. International Wound Journal. 2013;**10**:3-8

[7] Lese M, Micu-Chis RD. The microbiology of surgical infections. ResearchGate; January 2018. DOI: 10.30845/ ijast.v8n3p5

[8] Beisel WR. Overview of immune system and other host defense. In: Military Strategies for Sustainment of Nutrition and Immune Function in the Field. Washington, DC: National Academy Press; 1999. pp. 511-526

[9] Brightbill HD, Libraty DH, Krutzik SR, et al. Host defense mechanisms triggered by microbial lipoproteins through toll-like receptors. Science. 1999;**285**:732-736

[10] Accolla RS. Host defense mechanisms against pathogens. Surgical Infections. 2006;**7** (suppl. 2):S5-S7

[11] Dellinger RP, Schorr CA, Levy MM, et al. User's guide to the surviving sepsis guidelines. Critical Care Medicine. 2017;**45**:381-385

[12] Marik PE, Taeb AM. SIRS, qSOFA and new sepsis definition. Journal of Thoracic Disease. 2017;**9**:943-945

[13] Levy MM, Evans LE, Rhodes A, et al. The surviving sepsis campaign bundle: 2018 update. Critical Care Medicine. 2018;**46**:997-1000

Chapter 2

Immunoparalysis in Septic Shock Patients

Giorgio Berlot and Silvia Passero

Additional information is available at the end of the chapter

http://dx.doi.org/10.5772/intechopen.88866

Abstract

In the recent years, it has become clear that septic shock is characterized by the simultaneous production of inflammatory and anti-inflammatory mediators; the primary role of the latter is to counterbalance the former, thus limiting the severity of their systemic effects. However, in a number of patients, the anti-inflammatory substances can cause a downregulation in both the innate and adaptive immune capabilities, leading a second phase characterized to secondary infections caused by opportunist germs and the reactivation of latent viruses, muscle wasting; altogether, these abnormalities set the stage for a chronic critical condition. This condition, whose identification is relatively recent, is called immunoparalysis. Unfortunately, the current approach to septic shock is focused much more on the inflammatory phase than in the ensuing immunoparalysis, whose diagnosis can be challenging. In this chapter, the role played by both classes of mediators, the monitoring of the immune system, and the possible current and not yet available therapeutic strategies of immunoparalysis are reviewed and discussed.

Keywords: septic shock, compensatory anti-inflammatory reaction syndrome, immunoparalysis, immunomonitoring

1. Introduction

The classical clinical manifestations of septic shock (SS) include fever, tachycardia, arterial hypotension, and abnormalities of the white blood cell count (WBC) associated with a wide range of organ dysfunction carrying a substantial risk of death [1]; the current approach, issued under the auspices of the Surviving Sepsis Campaign on the basis of clinical trials fulfilling the evidence-based medicine (EBM) criteria, includes the rapid administration of wide-spectrum antibiotics, the maintenance of a proper perfusion pressure via the administration of fluids and/or to vasopressors, the drainage of septic foci, etc. [2]. Overall, it appears that both the description and the therapies apply to acutely ill patients suffering from an infection-induced overwhelming reaction determined by a huge number of pro-inflammatory mediators produced and released by the innate immunity system. However, more than 20 years ago, Bone [3] hypothesized that this early hyperinflammatory phase could be accompanied by a compensatory anti-inflammatory response (CARS) aiming to limit the tissue damage. In the last decade, the concept of CARS has changed from a time-limited and somehow beneficial mechanism to a harmful reaction, potentially leading to a condition of marked reduction of the immune capabilities known as immunoparalysis [4–6]. Clinically, this condition is marked by recurrent and/or unresolving infections caused by germs with relatively low virulence; the reactivation of silent virus such as *cytomegalovirus* (CMV), Epstein-Barr virus (EBV), and herpesvirus (HV); a persisting low-grade inflammation; nutrition-resistant hypercatabolism; and muscle wasting [7, 8] (**Table 1**). The immunoparalysis characterizes also the clinical course of the chronic critically ill patients, namely, subjects who survived the initial insult (i.e., septic shock due to pneumonia, peritonitis, etc.) but fails to recover enough to be weaned from the mechanical ventilation and discharged from the intensive care unit (ICU) [9]. Moreover it should be noted that factors other than pathophysiological mechanisms can reduce the immune response, including the administration of steroids and norepinephrine [1, 10]. The aims of this chapter are (1) to review the main mechanism determining a SS, (2) to describe the transition from an easily recognizable hyperinflammatory condition to a less straightforward diagnosable one featured by a downregulation of the immune capabilities, (3) to provide some monitoring tools of the immune function, and, finally, (4) to identify some possible therapeutic approaches.

Variable	Uncontrolled inflammatory response	Immunoparalysis
Clinical phenotype	Fever, arterial hypotension, elevated cardiac output, rapidly evolving MODS, community or surgical infections	Altered mental status, normo-/hypothermia, slow-evolving MODS, health care- or hospital-acquired infections
Patients population	Young, middle-aged	Elderly, fragile
Comorbidities	Often absent	Often present
	Low Charlson's index	High Charlson's index
Germs characteristics	Virulent, toxin releasing	Low virulence, opportunistic
		Latent virus reactivation
Laboratory findings	↑↑ or ↓ neutrophil count,	↓ lymphocyte
	↑ blood lactate levels	
Nutritional status	Normal	Sarcopenia/cachexia
		Muscle wasting
Clinical course	Resolution of sepsis	Protracted ICU LOS
	Immunorestoration	Chronic critical disease
	Early deaths	Late deaths

LOS, length of stay.

Table 1. Different clinical presentations of sepsis-induced immunological alterations.

2. Pathophysiology of septic shock: a classical overview

2.1. The inflammatory response

Since the late 1970s, it has become clear that the clinical and biochemical manifestations of sepsis and its related complications are not caused directly by invading germ(s) but rather by the host's response to the infection. The innate immune response largely accounts for the above described signs and symptoms. The presence of microorganism-derived substances collectively known as pathogen-associated molecular pattern (PAMP) which include endotoxin, capsular antigens, elements derived from the cell wall, flagellins, and other substances derived from the bacterial lysis determines the rapid activation of genes encoding for an extremely elevated (and still partially unknown) mediators able to trigger a strong inflammatory reaction, including the tumor necrosis factor-α (TNF), a number of interleukins (IL), the platelet-activating factor (PAF), etc. (**Table 2**). It is worthwhile to recall that (a) the list of mediators is incomplete because new elements are added on a weekly or at maximum monthly basis, (b) the rise of blood levels of inflammatory mediators is a matter of minutes since it represents the first line of defense to contrast the deleterious effects of PAMP and DAMPS, and (c) for this reason, the innate response is highly similar among all species of mammalians [6].

Independently from their biochemical structure, the term inflammasome lumps together all these heterogeneous mediators that are characterized by (a) the presence of many positive and negative feedback loops, determining an array that can be better conceived as a network

Cytokine	Source	Effects	Interactions	Antagonists
TNF	Innate and adaptive immune system	Activation of immune cells Fever cachexia, apoptosis	Activation of downstream inflammatory mediators	Soluble TNF receptors Anti-TNF ab
IL-1	"	Fever, pro-coagulation Hematopoiesis	"	IL-1 receptor antagonists
IL-6	"	Activation of T and B lymphocytes Fever	Inhibits the release of TNF and IL-1 Promotes anti-inflammatory response	IL-6 receptor antagonists
IL-12	Monocyte, macrophages, neutrophils, dendritic cells	Activation of adaptive response	Promotes IFN-γ production	Unknown
IFN-γ	NKT cells CD 8 T cell	Antiviral action Potentially reverse immunoparalysis	Released in response to TNF, IL-12, and IL-18	Unknown

TNF, tumor necrosis factor; IL, interleukin; IFN, interferon.

Table 2. Some relevant pro-inflammatory mediators.

and not a cascade, thus making understandable the therapeutic failure demonstrated in many trials in which septic patients were treated with substances aimed to the block a single mediator via monoclonal or chimeric specific antibodies (Ab) such as anti-TNFαAb or with the administration of circulating antagonists (ra) (i.e., soluble IL1-ra and TNF TNFα-ra) directed to block the receptors present on the cell surface; (b) the pleiotropic and paracrine effects, accounting for the multiple effects exerted in different organs; (c) the interference with the mitochondria causing a disturbance of the O_2 uptake and consumption by the tissues; and (d) the interaction with other biological systems including the complement system and the coagulative cascade. Notably, the very same mediators are produced in noninfectious conditions, including trauma, low-flow states, surgery, burns, etc.; in these circumstances the trigger is represented by an intracellular substance derived from the injured tissues (DAMP, damage-associated molecular patterns). The endothelium is massively involved in this reaction causing a microvascular plugging and the abnormal production of nitric oxide (NO) which exert a profound vasodilation [11, 12].

From an evolutionary perspective, it is likely that these mediators have been developed and maintained, aiming to contain the initial inoculum and to destroy the responsible organisms. This explains why in most cases an infection does not cause a SS: actually, the latter occurs only when the pro-inflammatory mediators exert their effects at a systemic level, thus determining the clinical phenotype of SS and the almost unavoidable presence of the simultaneous dysfunction of different organs and systems even not directly involved by the infection (MODS).

2.2. The compensatory reaction

The secretion of inflammasome is accompanied by the production of other substances aimed to limit their action at a local level and, at the same time, to prevent their systemic spread (**Table 3**). As stated above for the inflammatory mediators, their list is incomplete for the very same reasons. Actually, it was hypothesized that during the initial phase (almost), only pro-inflammatory mediators were produced and that these conditions subsided due to the action of the CARS-associated mediators. Despite its popularity, it became clear that this scheme represents an oversimplification as (a) both classes of substances are produced since the initial phase of sepsis albeit in different rates; (b) the action of anti-inflammatory mediators is responsible for the late-onset immunoparalysis; and finally (c) a low-level production of pro-inflammatory substances can be maintained even during the advanced stages of sepsis leading to malnutrition, protein waste, and reduced adaptive immunity. Overall, the sepsis-associated immunoparalysis resembles the normal aging process of the immune system (immunosenescence) that is characterized by the overall downregulation of both the innate and adaptive immunity functions. This appears particularly relevant as the ever-increasing age of septic patients exposes them to both conditions.

Put shortly, it appears that the mediators implicated in the CARS can represent a double-edged sword, as they both can exert (a) a beneficial role when they determine the restoration of the immune condition existing prior to the sepsis (immune restoration) and (b) can trigger a life-threatening condition when their excess production and/or duration of action causes the shutdown of the immune response [13, 14].

http://dx.doi.org/10.5772/intechopen.88866

Cytokine	Source	Effects	Interactions
IL-10	Innate and adaptive immune system	Immunosuppression Inhibition of antigen presentation and phagocytosis	Suppression of the production of inflammatory mediators
TGF-β	Macrophages Smooth muscle cells	Immunosuppression	"
IL-4	Mast cells T_h2 T cells Basophils Eosinophils	Promotes T_h2 T-cell differentiation	Induces the production of IL-10

TGF, transforming growth factor.

Table 3. Some relevant anti-inflammatory mediators.

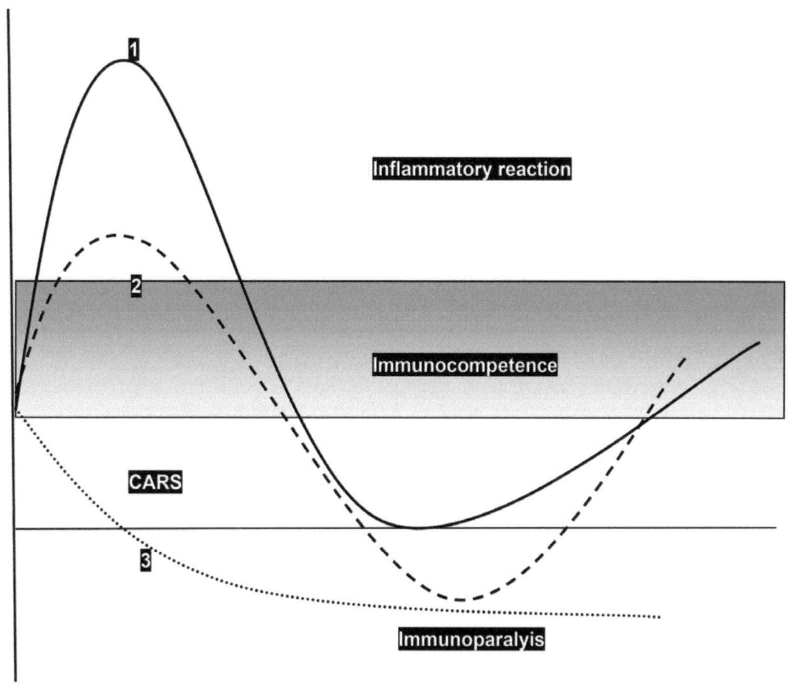

Figure 1. Possible clinical trajectories of patients with sepsis shock. Line 1, intense hyperinflammatory reaction followed by CARS and the return to the baseline immune state. Line 2, weak hyperinflammatory reaction followed by immunoparalysis and immune restoration. Line 3, immunoparalysis not preceded by a hyperinflammatory reaction.

In conclusion, (at least) three clinical trajectories can be hypothesized (**Figure 1**): the first includes patients with an intense hyperinflammatory reaction that subsides once the CARS is well established and the immune function is restored; in the second the initial phase is shorter and weaker, and the CARS determines a short-lived immunoparalysis preceding the return toward the baseline immune function; and in the third one, the CARS prevails and causes the loss of the immune capabilities.

3. The determinants of immunoparalysis

Only recently it became clear that the CARS does not represent only a physiologic counterbalance to the inflammatory response to PAMP and DAMP but that it can determine a critical condition in and by itself [13, 15].

Actually, different experimental and clinical studies indicate that the advanced stage of sepsis and SS is characterized by a reduction of both the innate and adaptive immune responses (**Table 4**). Extensive evidence supports this model, even if large inter-patient differences exist. First, monocytes present a reduced expression of membrane HLA-DR in association to either a decreased secretion of inflammatory mediators when stimulated or a diminished antigen presentation. Second, different membrane-bound receptors able to potentiate the immune response, including IL-2α, IL-7R α, CD86, etc., are reduced. Third, the production of immunosuppressant substances, such and programmed death 1 (PD1) and its ligand (PD-L1), is increased in antigen-presenting cells, thus inhibiting the activation of T lymphocytes. Fourth, there is an increased appearance of immunosuppressive T-cell subpopulations, such as myeloid-derived suppressor cell and $CD4^+$ and $CD25^+$ T-regulatory cells (T_{reg}), which suppress adaptive immunity. These appear to be particularly relevant, as Treg (a) actively produce anti-inflammatory cytokines including TGF-β and IL-10, (b) downregulate the secretion of pro-inflammatory mediators, (c)

Factors involved	Marker
Monocyte deactivation	↓ mHLA-DR expression
	↓ TNF-α production
Tissue macrophage dysfunction	Presently none
Negative regulatory mediators	↑ PD-(L)1 expression
	↑ CTL-4, BTLA expression
	↑ LAG-3 and TIM-3 expression
Receptors downregulation	↓ IL-7 receptor
Apoptosis	↑ FAS
	↓ lymphocytes
Suppression of immune cells	↑ CD-4, CD-25
	↑ myeloid-derived suppressor cells
Anti-inflammatory cytokines	↑ IL-10, IL-13, IL-4, IL1 receptor antagonists, TGF-β
	↑ IL-10/TNF-α

mHLA-DR, human leukocyte antigen on the monocyte surface; PD-(L1), programmed death ligand; CTLA-4, cytotoxic lymphocyte antigen 4; BTLA, B and T lymphocyte attenuator; LAG-3, lymphocyte activation gene 3; TIM-3, T lymphocyte immunoglobulin protein 3; sFAS, soluble FAS ligand; TGF-β, transforming growth factor-β.

Table 4. Factors of immunosuppression.

Mechanisms	Effect
Endotoxin tolerance	↑ Anti-inflammatory mediators, ↓ pro-inflammatory mediators
	↓ Antigen presentation
Apoptosis	↓ Immune cell number
	Immune cell number anergy
Energy failure	Immune cell anergy
	Apoptosis
Epigenetic regulation	↓ Pro-inflammatory mediators

Table 5. Mechanisms of immunoparalysis.

neutralize cytotoxic T cells, and (d) deactivate the monocytes. Fourth, immune cells present an increased apoptosis, and their loss is not replaced enough by the production of new ones. Finally, the phagocytosis of apoptotic cells by fixed and circulating macrophages leads to a switch of the latter to the M2 phenotype, whose feature is an increased production of the anti-inflammatory substances IL-10 and IL-1ra. Put briefly, all these mechanisms exert their action via relatively few common pathways, which include the increased apoptosis determining the reduction of immune cells, the loss of antigen presentation, the blunted response to PAMP, and the reduction of energy production caused by the impairment of the glucose metabolism (**Table 5**) [16, 17]. All these reactions are driven by epigenetic changes causing in different time frames the activation or deactivation of genes involved in the immune response, and the resulting phenotype is an intense inflammatory response or, conversely, an immunoparalysis.

4. The diagnosis of immunoparalysis

The recognition of sepsis-induced immunoparalysis is not straightforward because the clinical manifestations associated with the switch from the hyperinflammatory state to CARS and the full-blown depression of the immune capabilities are not so protean as the symptoms of SS [18]. Moreover, the SSC guidelines focus almost exclusively on the former and pay much less attention, if any, to the latter. From a practical and clinical point view, some issues appear particularly relevant.

4.1. Timing of onset

The transition from the hyperinflammatory phase to immunoparalysis can be challenging to identify and to monitor at the bedside and represents a kind of no man's land in the clinical course of patients which survived from the initial phase of SS.

The onset is highly variable. Actually, although the secretion of immunomodulatory substances can occur relatively early, their clinical consequences present wide variations. Some authors [19] observed a substantial difference of mHLA-DR starting from 3 to 7 days in a small group of surgical septic patients, and other authors demonstrated that significant decrease of the CD14/HLA-DR and of heat-shock proteins (HSP) 70 and 90 was present already within 24 hours from the onset of sepsis [5]; in both studies, these alterations were more marked in patients who developed SS later on. More recently, Morris et al. [20] in association with raised percentage of regulatory T cells (T_{reg}) were predictive for infections occurring between 3 and 9 days after ICU admission, and a similar timing has been demonstrated also in another study in which the mortally rate of secondary infection was ~14% [17]. On the basis of these findings, it is reasonable to hypothesize that (a) a combination of cellular and soluble factors able to blunt the immune response is present since the very initial phase of sepsis; (b) their effects on the clinical course, namely, the appearance of secondary infections and/or viral reactivation, can occur within the initial 10 days from the admission; and (c) these are associated with a substantial mortality of patients surviving the initial insult.

4.2. Monitoring of the immune function

In ICU patients, every organ system is monitored to allow a change in the treatment tailored on the variation observed. An ideal monitoring system should be accurate, cheap, and not labor-intensive, and the information gathered should be readily if not continuously available. Since it has become clear that the immune system in sepsis undergoes modifications not reflected by the commonly measured biological variables such as the arterial pressure, the heart rate, the urinary output, etc., different investigations aimed to identify one or more markers of changes of its functions whose follow-up could be valuable to modify the therapy according to its changes: as an example, the occurrence of immunoparalysis contraindicates the administration of steroids whose use is recommended by the SSC guidelines.

Several monitoring systems exploring both legs of the immune response have been developed so far, based on the repeated assessments of the cells involved, their response to different

Function	Cell	Marker	Outcome	Lab technique	Runaround (h)
Innate immunity	Neutrophils	↑ Immature forms	Death Secondary infections	FC. Hematology analyzer	1.5
	Monocytes	↓ HLA-DR	Death Secondary infections	FC, IHC, PCR	1.5
Adaptive immunity	All lymphocytes	Lymphopenia	Death Secondary infections	FC. Hematology analyzer	0.5
	White blood cells	NTL	Death Secondary infections	FC. Hematology analyzer	0.5
Both	Lymphocytes	Viral reactivation	Death	PCR	12

FC, flow cytometry; IHC, immunohistochemistry; PCR, polymerase chain reaction; NTL, neutrophil/lymphocyte ratio.

Table 6. Some currently available indicators of immune function.

challenges, and the measurement of the blood concentrations of soluble mediators involved in the different clinical frames [14, 15, 21, 22]. It could be useful to describe separately those currently available and those which will be used likely in the next future. Most of the former (**Table 6**) can be obtained cheaply and on a daily basis; among all, the neutrophil-to-lymphocyte ratio has been indicated as the less costly and more rapidly available monitoring tool [23, 24]. Other advanced, expensive, and not yet widely available monitoring tools take advantage of more sophisticated lab techniques (**Table 7**) requiring lab expertise and financial resources putting them at risk of not being used outside the research center. Another dynamic approach, which shares the very same limitations of the previously described advanced techniques, consists in challenging the immune cells with substances able to trigger their activation, including LPS, other PAMP, and phytohemoagglutinin; actually, a number of investigators demonstrated that a blunted response to the stimulation is associated with an increased rate of severe infectious complications in different patient populations [25–27].

Independently from the systems used, it should be clear that the monitoring of the immune response in septic as well in other clinical conditions (a) is based on the time variations of a panel of indicators and not on a single one and (b) due to their direct and indirect costs,

Function	Cell	Marker	Outcome	Lab technique	Runaround (h)
Innate immunity	Monocytes	↓ sCD127	Death, secondary infections	FC, PCR, IHC, ELISA	5
		Endotoxin tolerance	Not clear	Cell culture, ELISA, FC, IHC	72
		↑ PD-L1	Secondary infections	FC, IHC	1.5
		IL10/TNF ratio	Death	ELISA	5
	Dendritic cells	↓ Count	Death, secondary infections	FC	1.5
Adaptive immunity	All lymphocytes	↑ CTLA 4, BTLA	Not clear	FC, IHC	1.5
		↑ PD	Death	FC, IHC	1.5
		CD 127	Death, secondary infections	FC, IHC	1.5
	T cells	Proliferation	Death, secondary infections	Cell culture + FC	72
			MODS		
	T_{reg}	↑ T_{reg}	Death	FC	1.5
Both	Transcriptomic	CD 74, CX3CR1	Not clear	PCR, microarray	72

FC, flow cytometry; IHC, immunohistochemistry; PCR, polymerase chain reaction; ELISA, enzyme-linked immunosorbent assay.

Table 7. Some promising, yet not currently available, markers of immunoparalysis.

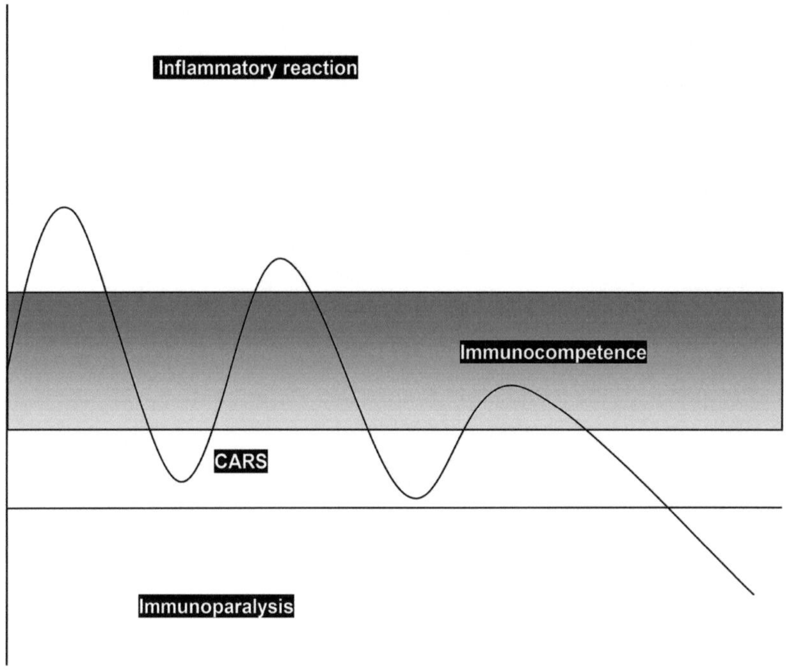

Figure 2. The multiple hits phenomenon ultimately leading to the exhaustion of the immune response.

it should be limited to the subjects at risk; as an example, it is worthwhile to monitor the immune function in patients undergoing multiple abdominal surgical procedures for suture dehiscence but not in another one safely recovering after peritonitis.

4.3. The identification of patients at risk of immunoparalysis

Even with the exclusion of clinical conditions and/or treatments known to cause an immunoparalysis (i.e., solid and hematologic cancers, autoimmune disorders), etc., this circumstance can occur in virtually all ICU patients; however, different studies identified some predisposing factors that should be considered particularly relevant, including septic shock, advanced age, health care-associated infections, elevated Charlson's score indicating a substantial underlying fragility, comorbidities, prolonged hospital and ICU length of stay, and multiple surgical procedures [17, 28, 29]. The latter, which are associated with the repeated activation of the inflammatory and anti-inflammatory responses, according to the multiple hits model, ultimately lead to the exhaustion of the immune response [30] (**Figure 2**).

5. The treatment of immunoparalysis

In the last decade, a number of drugs have been developed to restore a normal immune function in patients with solid or hematologic tumors on the basis of many investigations demonstrating the tumor cells are able to suppress in many different ways the host's immune response against themselves. Independently from the substance use and the molecular target, these innovative treatments have been demonstrated to be effective but somehow difficult to handle, as they are associated with a number of side effects ranging from mild to life-threatening [31]. As several similarities exist between tumor- and sepsis-induced blunting of the immune response [32], it is likely that in the next future the immune-boosting treatments will be developed to treat the latter, aiming to develop a precision medicine also in ICU patients [33] (**Table 8**).

Presently, according to the SSC guidelines [2], the immune-targeted approaches are limited to the administration of steroids in not fluid and catecholamine-responding SS, whereas the use of intravenous immunoglobulins (IvIg) is discouraged. Actually, this latter position is questionable as a number of trials performed in several thousands of patients demonstrated that (a) the administration of IvIg is associated with the reduction of mortality in different subsets of SS patients; (b) among the different preparations available, the only ones containing supra-normal concentrations of IgM and IgA appears more effective, and (c) the improvement of survival is time-dependent, as a ~6% increase of mortality has been observed for every day of delay in the administration [34].

Besides steroids and IvIg, other treatments aimed to modulate the immune response include blood purification (BPT) techniques and a number of substances able to boost it.

Cells/factors involved	Alterations	Possible therapies
Myeloid cells	↑ Immature neutrophils	GM-CSF
	↑ Tolerant dendritic cells	Toll-like receptor antagonists
	↑ Myeloid-derived suppressor cells	FTL3L
	↓ Monocyte HLA-DR expression	TNF
Lymphocytes	↓ Cytokine production	Anti-PD1 ab
	Altered metabolism	Anti-PDL 1 ab
	↓ Proliferation	Anti CTLA4, TIM3, LAG3 ab
	↑ Immune checkpoint inhibitors	
	Malfunction of NKT cells	
	↑ T_{reg} and B_{reg} cells	
	↑ CD 155 expression	
↑ Systemic cytokine release	↑ IL-10	GM-CSF
	↑ PGE 2	TLR agonists
	↑ TGFβ	FT3L
		TNF

GMC-SF, granulocyte-macrophage colony-stimulating factor; FTL3L, FMS-related tyrosine kinase 3 ligand; PD, programmed death; PDL1, programmed cell death ligand 1; CTL4, cytotoxic T-cell protein 4; TIM3, T-cell immunoglobulin mucin receptor 3; T_{reg} B_{reg}, regulatory T and B cells; TGFβ, transforming growth factor-β; PGE, prostaglandin E2.

Table 8. Immunosuppressive pathways shared by cancer and sepsis.

5.1. Blood purification techniques

Since the 1980s, a number of extracorporeal techniques have been developed aiming to remove the "toxic" mediators responsible for the clinical manifestations of SS.

Independently from their principle of functioning (see later), the BPT consists in an extracorporeal circuit where the patient's blood flows till enters in the depurative device; once the latter is passed, the blood returns to the patient. According to the principle used, the BPT can be subdivided into (a) blood processing or (b) plasma processing techniques. In the former, the whole blood is depurated via a number techniques, which differ in terms of type and surface of the membranes used, their permeability to the high molecular weight of the septic mediators, etc., whereas in the latter the plasma is separated from the blood, processed in a cartridge, and reinfused downstream. The mediators can be eliminated through the membranes or adsorbed over it. In both cases, the neutralizing capabilities are time-limited. A detailed description of the BPT is beyond the aim of this chapter, but some considerations are necessary. First, there are no studies clearly demonstrating the superiority of one of them, even if some meta-analysis indicates that the those using the adsorption are more effective; (b) they can remove also antibiotics, nutrients, vitamins, hormones, etc.; (c) they require anticoagulation; and, most importantly; and (d) they are not selective and thus remove pro- as well as anti-inflammatory mediators [35].

5.2. Immune-boosting agents

Different substances have been used or likely will be used in the next future (**Table 9**) to enhance the depressed immune function in septic and non-septic critically ill patients, including [36, 37]:

- **Interferon-γ** (**IFN-γ**) is a cytokine produced by helper T cell and an activator of monocytes. Different case series and case report performed in a limited number of patients demonstrated that its administration was associated with an increased HLA-DR expression; however, presently there are no RCT fulfilling the EBM criteria demonstrating a beneficial effect on the outcome of patients with SS.
- **Granulocyte-macrophage colony-stimulating factor** (**GMC-SF**) stimulates the production of neutrophils from the bone marrow. Even if prophylactic use in neutropenic patients did not demonstrate any beneficial effect, a number of investigations demonstrated that its administration was associated with an improved outcome especially in patients with a decreased HLA-DR expression.
- **Interleukin-7** (**IL-7**) is a cytokine released by bone marrow and thymus cells that prompts the growth and the differentiation of T cells. This substance is considered an immune-boosting agent in patients with cancer and multifocal leukoencephalopathy and in septic patients suffering from immunoparalysis.
- **Programmed death inhibitors** (**PD1i**) are proteins whose effect is to block the programmed death of immune cells, which appears to be a critical factor for the progression of cancer.

	Treatment	Effect	Pro	Against
Available	IvIg	Antibacterial action ↓ TNF and other pro-inflammatory mediators	Many small RCT demonstrated their efficacy	No EBM-validated Heterogeneity of patients treated High costs
	Blood purification techniques	Removal of mediators	Many small RCT demonstrated their efficacy	Not selective Heterogeneity of techniques (i.e., HVHV vs. plasma adsorption) Heterogeneity of patients treated Need of anticoagulation Not selective
Not yet available	Interferon-γ	Enhanced production of pro-inflammatory mediators	Some small RCT and case reports demonstrated its efficacy	Possible septic shock-like Systemic inflammatory reactions
	GMC-SF	Enhanced production of immune cells	"	Possible septic shock-like Systemic inflammatory reactions
	IL-7	Enhanced production of pro-inflammatory mediators	"	Possible septic shock-like Systemic inflammatory reactions
	Immune checkpoint inhibitors	Reduced apoptosis	"	Potentially severe and life-threatening side effects High costs No RCT available

Table 9. Possible immunomodulating treatments in septic shock.

This approach is new as it is aims to increase the immune response to the cancer cells without interfering with their metabolism. Due to their mechanism of action, their administration could determine a potentially life-threatening inflammatory reaction caused by the sudden release of mediators determining a "cytokine storm"; although their use is not codified yet in critically ill septic patients, in a recent RCT, the restoration of the immune response in the absence of a hyperinflammatory reaction was demonstrated in some SS patients given a novel PD1i at different doses [38].

6. Conclusions

Independently from its source, septic shock can be considered a double-step process: the initial phase is characterized by an intense inflammatory response that is counterbalanced by the production of several anti-inflammatory substances aiming to restore the immunity pre-sepsis steady state. However, in many cases this compensatory mechanism prevails and not only extinguishes the initial response but determines a condition of immunoparalysis that dominates the clinical course and influences the outcome. Unfortunately, the current approach is mainly directed against the initial inflammatory phase although some techniques of monitoring of the immune function are currently developed and others are being studied. The same concepts apply to treatments directed to potentiate the immune capabilities, but in this case the goal appears to be still far.

Author details

Giorgio Berlot* and Silvia Passero

*Address all correspondence to: berlot@inwind.it

Department of Anesthesia and Intensive Care, University of Trieste, Cattinara Hospital, Trieste, Italy

References

[1] Singer M, Deutschman CS, Seymour CW, et al. The third international consensus definitions for Sepsis and septic shock (sepsis-3). Journal of the American Medical Association. 2016;**315**(8):801-810. DOI: 10.1001/jama.2016.0287

[2] Rhodes A, Evans LE, Alhazzani W, et al. Surviving sepsis campaign: International guidelines for management of sepsis and septic shock: 2016. Intensive Care Medicine. 2017;**43**(3):304-377. DOI: 10.1007/s00134-017-4683-6

[3] Bone RC. Sir isaac newton, sepsis, SIRS, and CARS. Critical Care Medicine. 1996;**24**(7): 1125-1128

[4] Hotchkiss RS, Monneret G, Payen D. Immunosuppression in sepsis: A novel understanding of the disorder and a new therapeutic approach. The Lancet Infectious Diseases. 2013;**13**(3):260-268. DOI: 10.1016/S1473-3099(13)70001-X

[5] Papadopoulos P, Pistiki A, Theodorakopoulou M, et al. Immunoparalysis: Clinical and immunological associations in SIRS and severe sepsis patients. Cytokine. 2017;**92**:83-92. DOI: 10.1016/j.cyto.2017.01.012

[6] Ryan T, Coakley JD, Martin-Loeches I. Defects in innate and adaptive immunity in patients with sepsis and health care associated infection. Annals of Translational Medicine. 2017;**5**(22):447. DOI: 10.21037/atm.2017.09.21

[7] Horiguchi H, Loftus TJ, Hawkins RB, et al. Innate immunity in the persistent inflammation, immunosuppression, and catabolism syndrome and its implications for therapy. Frontiers in Immunology. 2018;**9**:595. DOI: 10.3389/fimmu.2018.00595

[8] Walton AH, Muenzer JT, Rasche D, et al. Reactivation of multiple viruses in patients with sepsis. PLoS One. 2014;**9**(6):e98819. DOI: 10.1371/journal.pone.0098819

[9] Stortz JA, Murphy TJ, Raymond SL, et al. Evidence for persistent immune suppression in patients who develop chronic critical illness after sepsis. Shock. 2018;**49**(3):249-258. DOI: 10.1097/SHK.0000000000000981

[10] Stolk RF, van der Poll T, Angus DC, et al. Potentially inadvertent immunomodulation: Norepinephrine use in Sepsis. American Journal of Respiratory and Critical Care Medicine. 2016;**194**(5):550-558. DOI: 10.1164/rccm.201604-0862CP

[11] Delano MJ, Ward PA. The immune System's role in Sepsis progression, resolution and long-term outcome. Immunological Reviews. 2016;**274**(1):330-353. DOI: 10.1111/imr.12499

[12] Schulte W, Bernhagen J, Bucala R. Cytokines in sepsis: Potent immunoregulators and potential therapeutic targets—An updated view. Mediators of Inflammation. 2013:16. DOI: 10.1155/2013/165974. Article ID 165974

[13] Hamers L, Kox M, Pickkers P. Sepsis-induced immunoparalysis: Mechanisms, markers, and treatment options. Minerva Anestesiologica. 2015;**81**(4):426-439

[14] Rouget C, Girardot T, Textoris J, et al. Biological markers of injury-induced immunosuppression. Minerva Anestesiologica. 2017;**83**(3):302-314. DOI: 10.23736/S0375-9393.16.11268-4

[15] Venet F, Monneret G. Advances in the understanding and treatment of sepsis-induced immunosuppression. Nature Reviews Nephrology. 2018;**14**(2):121-137. DOI: 10.1038/nrneph.2017.165

[16] Venet F, Lukaszewicz A-C, Payen D, et al. Monitoring the immune response in sepsis: A rational approach to administration of immunoadjuvant therapies. Current Opinion in Immunology. 2013;**25**(4):477-483. DOI: 10.1016/j.coi.2013.05.006

[17] van Vught LA, Klein Klouwenberg PMC, Spitoni C, et al. Incidence, risk factors, and attributable mortality of secondary infections in the intensive care unit after admission for sepsis. Journal of the American Medical Association. 2016;**315**(14):1469-1479. DOI: 10.1001/jama.2016.2691

[18] Pène F, Pickkers P, Hotchkiss RS. Is this critically ill patient immunocompromised? Intensive Care Medicine. 2016;**42**(6):1051-1054. DOI: 10.1007/s00134-015-4161-y

[19] Wu JF, Ma J, Chen J, et al. Changes of monocyte human leukocyte antigen-DR expression as a reliable predictor of mortality in severe sepsis. Critical Care. 2011;**15**(5):R220. DOI: 10.1186/cc10457

[20] Morris AC, Datta D, Shankar-Hari M, et al. Cell-surface signatures of immune dysfunction risk-stratify critically ill patients: INFECT study. Intensive Care Medicine. 2018;**44**(5):627-635. DOI: 10.1007/s00134-018-5247-0

[21] Fang W-F, Douglas IS, Chen Y-M, et al. Development and validation of immune dysfunction score to predict 28-day mortality of sepsis patients. PLoS One. 2017;**12**(10):e0187088. DOI: 10.1371/journal.pone.0187088

[22] Almansa R, Wain J, Tamayo E, et al. Immunological monitoring to prevent and treat sepsis. Critical Care. 2013;**17**:109. DOI: 10.1186/cc11922

[23] Hwang SY, Shin TG, Jo IJ, et al. Neutrophil-to-lymphocyte ratio as a prognostic marker in critically-ill septic patients. American Journal of Emergency Medicine. 2017;**35**(2):234-239. DOI: 10.1016/j.ajem.2016.10.055

[24] Salciccioli JD, Marshall DC, Pimentel MAF, et al. The association between the neutrophil-to-lymphocyte ratio and mortality in critical illness: An observational cohort study. Critical Care. 2015;**19**:13. DOI: 10.1186/s13054-014-0731-6

[25] Rol ML, Venet F, Rimmele T, et al. The REAnimation low immune status markers (REALISM) project: A protocol for broad characterisation and follow-up of injury-induced immunosuppression in intensive care unit (ICU) critically ill patients. BMJ Open. 2017;**7**(6):e015734. DOI: 10.1136/bmjopen-2016-015734

[26] Arens C, Kramm T, Decker S, et al. Association of immune cell subtypes and phenotype with subsequent invasive candidiasis in patients with abdominal sepsis. Shock. 2019;**52**(2):191-197. DOI: 10.1097/SHK.0000000000001251

[27] Dolin HH, Papadimos TJ, Stepkowski S, et al. A novel combination of biomarkers to herald the onset of Sepsis prior to the manifestation of symptoms. Shock. 2018;**49**(4):364-370. DOI: 10.1097/SHK.0000000000001010

[28] Sauaia A, Moore FA, Moore EE. Postinjury inflammation and organ dysfunction. Critical Care Clinics. 2017;**33**(1):167-191. DOI: 10.1016/j.ccc.2016.08.006

[29] Rivers EP, Jaehne AK, Nguyen HB, et al. Early biomarker activity in severe sepsis and septic shock and a contemporary review of immunotherapy trials: Not a time to give up, but to give it earlier. Shock. 2013;**39**(2):127-137. DOI: 10.1097/SHK.0b013e31827dafa7

[30] Lasanianos NG, Kanakaris NK, Dimitriou R, et al. Second hit phenomenon: Existing evidence of clinical implications. Injury. 2011;**42**(7):617-629. DOI: 10.1016/j.injury.2011.02.011

[31] Kroschinsky F, Stölzel F, von Bonin S, et al. New drugs, new toxicities: Severe side effects of modern targeted and immunotherapy of cancer and their management. Critical Care. 2017;**21**(1):89. DOI: 10.1186/s13054-017-1678-1

[32] Hotchkiss RS, Moldawer LL. Parallels between cancer and infectious disease. New England Journal of Medicine. 2014;**371**(4):380-383. DOI: 10.1056/NEJMcibr1404664

[33] Van Ton AMP, Kox M, Abdo WF, et al. Precision immunotherapy for sepsis. Frontiers in Immunology. 2018;**9**:1926. DOI: 10.3389/fimmu.2018.01926

[34] Berlot G, Vassallo MC, Busetto N, et al. Effects of the timing of administration of IgM- and IgA-enriched intravenous polyclonal immunoglobulins on the outcome of septic shock patients. Annals of Intensive Care. 2018;**8**:122. DOI: 10.1186/s13613-018-0466-7

[35] Ankawi G, Neri M, Zhang J, et al. Extracorporeal techniques for the treatment of critically ill patients with sepsis beyond conventional blood purification therapy: The promises and the pitfalls. Critical Care. 2018;**22**:262. DOI: 10.1186/s13054-018-2181-z

[36] Leentjens J, Kox M, van der Hoeven JG, et al. Immunotherapy for the adjunctive treatment of sepsis: From immunosuppression to immunostimulation. Time for a paradigm change? American Journal of Respiratory and Critical Care Medicine. 2013;**187**(12):1287-1293. DOI: 10.1164/rccm.201301-0036CP

[37] Venet F, Rimmelé T, Monneret G. Management of sepsis-induced immunosuppression. Critical Care Clinics. 2018;**34**(1):97-106. DOI: 10.1016/j.ccc.2017.08.007

[38] Hotchkiss RS, Colston E, Yende S, et al. Immune checkpoint inhibition in Sepsis: A phase 1b randomized, placebo-controlled, single ascending dose study of Antiprogrammed cell death-ligand 1 antibody (BMS-936559)*. Critical Care Medicine. 2019;**47**(5):632-642. DOI: 10.1097/CCM.0000000000003685

Chapter 3

Microbiota-Oriented Diagnostics and Therapy in Sepsis: Utopia or Necessity?

Ekaterina Chernevskaya and Natalia Beloborodova

Additional information is available at the end of the chapter

http://dx.doi.org/10.5772/intechopen.89187

Abstract

When diagnosing sepsis, it is common to look for pathogens, microbe's DNA, lipopolysaccharide (LPS), or host biomarkers while missing out on microbiota. The next-generation sequencing of 16S rRNA gene allowed characterizing the gut microbiota taxonomy and clarifying the gut microbial population being more complex than was previously thought. We suppose that significant disruption of the microbiota is an indicator of the major role it plays in sepsis. Serious metabolic disorders of the gut microbiota may contribute to an unfavorable outcome in septic patients. With the changes not only in the composition but also in the metabolic activity of the gut microbiota taken into account, the characteristics of the mechanisms of interactions in the "septic" microbiome will allow the advances in the optimization of the diagnostics and therapy of sepsis to be made.

Keywords: sepsis, gut microbiome, critical states, aromatic microbial metabolites, metabolome, organ dysfunction

1. Introduction

In recent years, the microbiome has been considered as an important player in the pathophysiology of various types of diseases, including trauma and sepsis [1, 2]. Over 70% of species of microorganisms are nonculturable and cannot be isolated as a pure culture for identification. Omics technologies (genomics, transcriptomics, metagenomic sequencing, proteomics, and metabolomics) have fully changed our concepts about the composition and function of the "invisible organ" [3]. Widespread distribution of microbiomic studies became possible about 10 years ago with the emergence of high-performance new-generation sequencing (NGS), allowing transcribing in mass the collective genome of microbiomes—metagenome. The 16S rRNA gene encodes highly specific RNA of bacterial ribosomes and is present in genomes of all known microorganisms. Its structure is quite conservative, but variable-specific regions allow identifying microorganisms of different species and strains. The study pattern is quite simple but rather laborious: at the first stage, DNA is isolated from a sample, and then a so-called genome library containing copies of gene 16S rRNA belonging to different bacteria is obtained. The library is "read" using high-performance sequenators providing reception of several thousand nucleotide sequences of gene 16S rRNA for each sample. The next stage deals with analysis of a huge body of received data using bioinformatic techniques. Results are represented in a way most suitable in each particular case. The introduction of latest technologies, for example, nanopore sequencing, allows fast identification of bacteria in samples and finding markers of resistance to antimicrobial drugs within 5–10 minutes with the portable real-time device for DNA and RNA sequencing "MinION" that weighs less than 100 grams. This method is currently undergoing clinical testing [4]. However, in a typical microbiome experiment, several aspects of microbial communities still remain inaccessible. These include low-abundance but potentially crucial taxa whose genetic material is not sampled by sequencing techniques due to being present below the level of detection [5]. The real value of all this novel knowledge to understand the pathogenesis of sepsis has yet to be established. In this chapter, we are discussing the important role of bacterial metabolites in comparison with taxonomic structure of the septic gut microbiota.

2. The gap between healthy and septic gut microbiomes

Sepsis is a multifaceted host response to an infecting pathogen that may be significantly amplified by endogenous factors [6]. The broader perspective also emphasizes the significant biological and clinical heterogeneity in affected individuals such as their age, underlying comorbidities, concurrent injuries (including surgery) and medications, and source of infection adding to further complexity [7]. The success of antibiotic treatment depends on rapid and accurate identification of relevant pathogens and is complicated by the increasing rate of antimicrobial resistance conditioned by the dynamic changes in the bacterial population in which aerobic and facultative anaerobic bacteria predominant at the onset of sepsis are replaced by anaerobic species as the oxygen levels deplete. Broad-spectrum therapy is administered in the absence of bacterial identification, but this may not accurately reflect causative pathogens [8].

For a better understanding of how to treat, we probably should change the paradigm from "anthropocentrism" to "microbiocentrism," as we think.

The presence of over hundreds of species in the gut of a healthy adult host is a way to survive in an ever-changing world and the ability to receive energy from different sources of food. In critical condition, the advantage is obtained by those species that are capable of surviving in more extreme conditions with less oxygen and a lack of nutrients and trace elements. For example, *Enterococcus* is one of the few microorganisms capable of surviving and thriving in the presence of bile acids, an increased concentration (6.5%) of NaCl, hydrogen peroxide, and changes in the pH level [9]. The most frequent cause of abdominal sepsis is a leakage of fecal material from the intestinal lumen into the peritoneal cavity [10]. The leakage introduces gut bacteria, including *Enterobacteriaceae, Enterococcus* spp., *Streptococcus* spp., and *Staphylococcus* spp., into the sterile peritoneal environment. Another prospective study of 32 patients admitted to the ICU after the trauma and acute care surgery service similarly found a replacement of intestinal *Faecalibacterium* and *Ruminococcus* with the more pathogenic *Enterococcus* [11]. The site of infection is not usually in the gut, but the metabolic influence of the pathogens on the gut microbiota and host tends to be persistently overlooked. For example, microbes that flourished in the guts of elite athletes boosted the time that lab mice ran on a treadmill. These particular microbes seem to take lactate, pumped out by muscles during exercise, and turn it into a compound that may contribute to endurance [12].

In our preliminary study, we used gas chromatography-mass spectrometry (GC-MS) analysis of blood serum and feces simultaneously and at the same time analyzed the taxonomic composition of the gut microbiota using 16S rRNA gene-based metagenomic analysis in groups of patients with sepsis, $n = 9$, and healthy, $n = 5$. The sepsis was diagnosed according to the Sepsis 3 definition [7].

The taxonomic composition of the gut microbiota in a group at the phylum level as determined by the metagenomic analysis of feces is shown in **Figure 1**. The major four phyla of the human gut microbiota, *Bacteroidetes, Firmicutes, Proteobacteria, Actinobacteria,* were the predominant phyla in most patients. The composition of the gut microbiota was not stable in any of the patients, and dynamic changes were observed in all nine patients. At the same time, the absolute percentage of *Proteobacteria* in septic patients was several times higher than in healthy volunteers. This was confirmed at the family level. The *Enterobacteriaceae* family, which is a part of the *Proteobacteria,* was shown to represent the leading species among the top 10 in sepsis. However, clear understanding cannot be reached using only taxonomy since it allows to observe only a handful of processes taking place in the development of any infection (**Figure 1**).

As we have shown earlier, high levels of some aromatic microbial metabolites (AMMs) in serum are related to the severity and mortality of critically ill patients [13]. The sum of the level of eight most relevant metabolites, benzoic (BA), phenylpropionic (PhPA), phenyllactic (PhLA), p-hydroxyphenylbenzoic (p-HBA), p-hydroxyphenylacetic (p-HPhAA), p-hydroxyphenylpropionic (p-HPhPA), homovanillic (HVA), and p-hydroxyphenyllactic acids (p-HPhLA), in serum samples from septic patients was higher than in healthy people 3.7 (1.2–8.0) μM and 1.3 (1.0–1.6) μM, respectively ($p < 0.05$). In the septic group, the maximum values of the sum of these metabolites were more than 10 μM which is higher than in patients with lethal outcome. The differences in the AMM quality profiles of simultaneously serum and fecal samples (SFS) of patients with sepsis and healthy are presented in **Figure 2**. The results showed that the feces of healthy people abound with such metabolites, p-PhAA, p-HPhPA, and p-HPhLA, supporting data obtained by Jenner et al. [14]. At the same time, we observed prevalence of BA, PhLA, and p-PhAA in sepsis with a higher level of BA in the gut of non-survivors. Differences in the proportion of AMM in the blood compared to the intestine can be explained by the fact that most hydrophilic (p-HPhAA, p-HPhLA, and PhLA) metabolites are excreted by the kidneys, while lipophilic metabolites (BA, PhAA, and PhPA) are absorbed by cells of tissue barriers (intestinal wall, lymphoid tissue, liver, vascular endothelium, etc.).

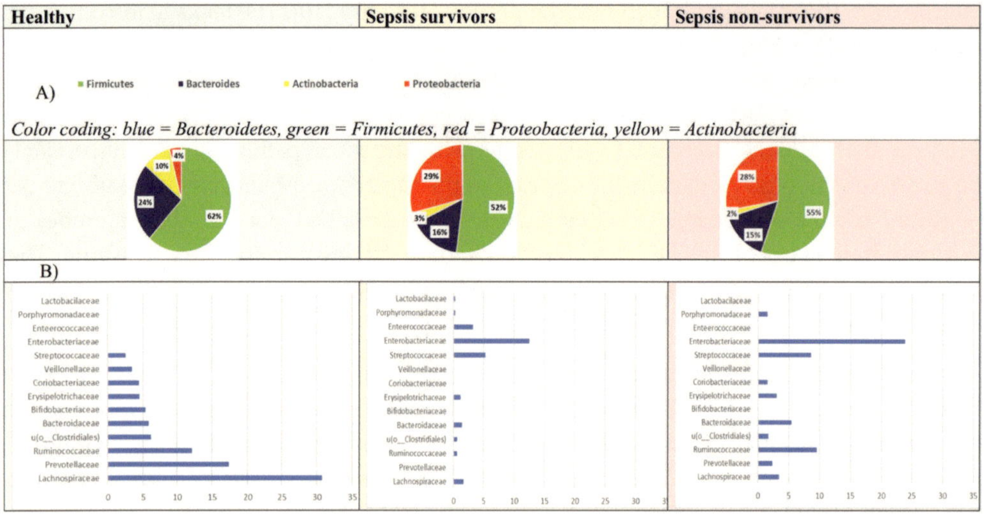

Figure 1. Taxonomic composition of the gut microbiota by metagenomic analysis. Comparison the taxonomic composition of the gut microbiota: (a) at the major phylum and (b) by top 10 families.

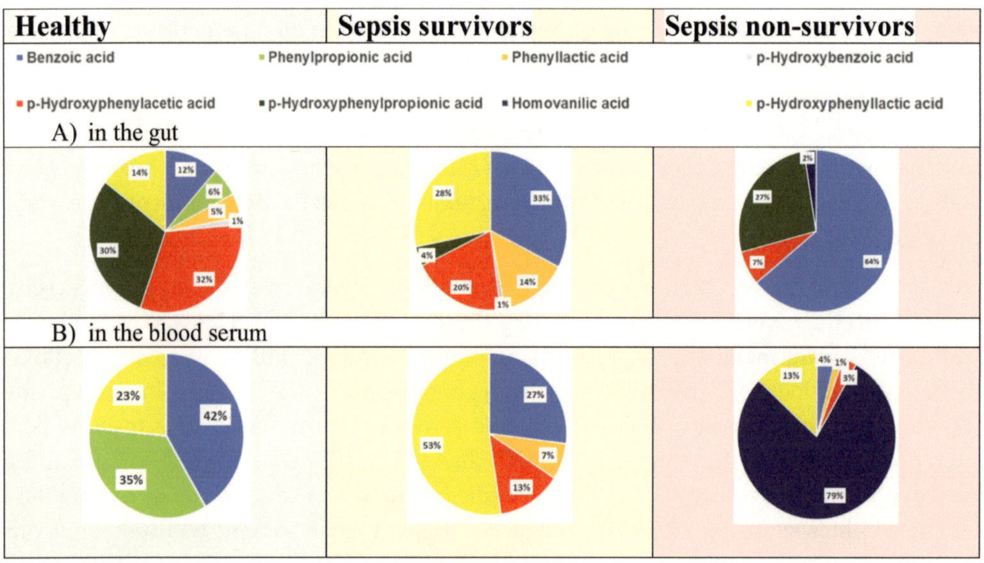

Figure 2. Metabolic profile of aromatic metabolites in: (A) the gut and (B) the blood serum. The data are presented by median of the proportion of each acid among all AMMs.

In particular, serum samples of healthy people are characterized by a predominance of BA and PhPA, while hydrophilic AMMs are detected in sepsis with the appearance of high levels of HVA in the serum of non-survivors. BA is a product of the synthesis of bacteria, plants, and fungi, but a significant content is formed as a result of biodegradation of phenylalanine.

Experimental study of the proximal part of the gastrointestinal tract showed that BA had a bacteriostatic and bactericidal dose-dependent effect on coliform and lactic acid bacteria [15].

On the one hand, it is important to emphasize that the dysfunction of the microbiota is manifested by excessive production of certain microbial metabolites as a reflection of the high microbial load with pathological colonization by bacteria involved in the development of sepsis. On the other hand, microbiota function, which is very important for host homeostasis, such as microbial biodegradation of an excess of endogenous biologically active compounds, due to a decrease in biodiversity in the intestine, primarily a deficiency of indigenous anaerobes, is disturbed [16]. The altered profile of aromatic metabolites in the blood may be an integral indicator reflecting these dramatic disturbances and possibly other functions of the "invisible organ."

3. The gut microbial metabolites in the pathogenesis of sepsis

It was shown that in vitro some sepsis-associated AMM in clinically significant concentrations can inhibit the phagocytic activity of neutrophils [17]; cause mitochondrial dysfunction [18]; influence on platelet aggregation [19]; reduce tyrosine hydroxylase activity, thus limiting the synthesis of catecholamines; and participate in the pathogenesis of septic shock [20]. Numerous data obtained in vitro allow us to hypothesize that AMM acts as signaling molecules (**Figure 3**).

It is impossible to exclude the presence of common signaling pathways, cell receptors, transmembrane transporters, and other mechanisms of humans and bacteria, as well as the direct participation of microbial metabolites in the pathogenesis of sepsis. Thus, today, we should not confine ourselves to studying eukaryotic cells while searching for new molecular mechanisms of sepsis-associated organ failure and septic shock [20]. We should consider

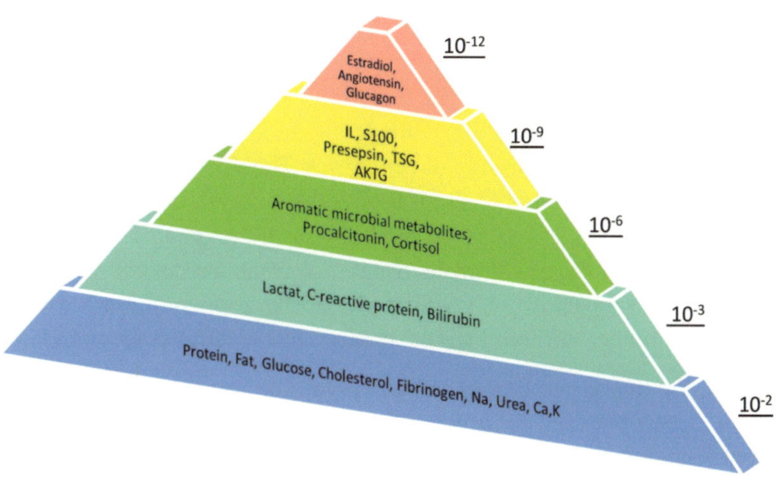

Figure 3. Schematic representation of levels of some biochemical parameters, metabolites, and hormones in blood serum in comparison.

and simulate experimental changes in the internal environment of a person that occur with a radical "restructuring" of the microbiome in seriously ill patients. This approach opens new prospects for an objective monitoring of diseases, carrying out an assessment of the integral metabolic profile on common metabolites (particularly aromatic) within a given time, and will provide new targets for therapeutic effects in the future.

4. Microbiome-oriented therapy: how to keep balance?

In sepsis, disturbances of physiological parameters caused directly by patient's conditions and multiple treatment-induced factors might have powerful impact on the gut microbiome. Finding a therapy aimed at restoring the balance between "beneficial" and "harmful" microorganisms is highly relevant. At present, there are several possible approaches (**Table 1**):

- Increase the "beneficial" microorganisms using pro-, pre-, and/or metabiotics.
- Use a combination of probiotics and prebiotics known as symbiotics.
- Improve the composition by transplantation of fecal microbiota transplantation (FMT).
- Suppress "harmful" microorganisms, and create favorable conditions for recovery of one's own "beneficial" microorganisms using selective antibacterial drugs (similar selective digestive decontamination).

The undoubtful effectiveness of probiotics for correction of functional disorders of the gastrointestinal tract has been widely accepted. A randomized placebo-controlled study on 4556 healthy newborns in India proved that oral probiotics *Lactobacillus plantarum* combined with fructo-oligosaccharides during the first postnatal week helped reduce sepsis incidence during the first 60 days of life [21]. A randomized, double-blind, placebo-controlled, experimental study of changes in the microbiome and intestinal barrier in early sepsis showed that probiotic intervention successfully modulates the microbiome and is therefore a promising tool for early intervention in sepsis [22]. At the same time, there are no recommendations for the use of probiotics in ICU yet. Present studies differ due to the diseases in patients, the microorganism strains used, and the prescribed dosage of probiotics. There is no consensus concerning the beginning and duration of treatment. As for today, the largest study of efficacy of probiotics and symbiotics in ICU patients was carried out by Manzanares et al. The sample of over 2700 patients demonstrated that the use of probiotics for microbiota recovery reduced incidence of infectious complications (specifically, ventilation-associated pneumonias); it was possible to reduce the use of antibiotics without increasing mortality or length of stay in ICU [23].

In another study, the use of symbiotics as an adjuvant therapy in surgical patients reduced incidence of such postoperative complications as wound infection [24]. One of the reasons for doubts concerning expediency of applying probiotics in ICU is intestinal barrier failure in critically ill patients. The translocation of bacteria to systemic blood flow and lymph is known to promote a complex chain of events leading to multiple organ failure [34]. On this

http://dx.doi.org/10.5772/intechopen.89187

	Study	Population	Type of intervention	Results
Probiotics/symbiotics				
☺	Panigrahi et al. [21]	4556 healthy newborns	*Lactobacillus plantarum*	Reduction in the incidence of sepsis during the first 60 days of life
☺	Stadlbauer et al. [22]	15 patients with early sepsis	The multispecies probiotic in a dose of 10^9 daily	Probiotic intervention successfully modulates the microbiome
☺	Manzanares et al. [23]	Meta-analysis of 30 trials that enrolled 2972 critically ill patients	Different types of probiotic therapy	Probiotics were associated with a significant reduction in infections (risk ratio 0.80, 95% confidence interval (CI) 0.68, 0.95, P = 0.009; heterogeneity I2 = 36%, P = 0.09)
☺	Kasatpibal et al. [24]	Meta-analysis of 31 articles that enrolled 2952 surgical patients	Different types of probiotic, prebiotic and symbiotic therapy	Symbiotic therapy was the best regimen in reducing surgical site infection (SSI) (RR = 0.28; 95% CI, 0.12–0.64)
☺	Besselink et al. [25]	298 patients with predicted severe acute pancreatitis	4 species of lactic bacterial (*L. acidophilus, L. casei, L. salivarius, L. lactis*), and 2 species of bifid bacteria (*B. bifidum, B. lactis*) in a dose of 10^{10} daily	Probiotic prophylaxis is associated with an increased risk of mortality and higher rate of infectious complications
FMT				
☺	Han et al. [26]	Review of management of *Clostridium difficile* infection (CDI) with a focus on FMT	FMT	The potential effective therapy but not enough data in the ICU patients
☺	Moayyedi et al. [27]	Meta-analysis of 5 trials that enrolled 284 patients with CDI	FMT (including autologous FMT)	FMT was statistically significantly more effective (RR, 0.41; 95% CI, 0.22–0.74; NNT, 3; 95% CI, 2–7) than vancomycin or placebo
☺	McClave et al. [28]	Review of clinical use of fecal microbial transplantation in critical illness	FMT	An attractive option to mitigate multiple organ dysfunction in the ICU
☺	FDA [29]	Two immunocompromised patients	FMT	The development of a severe infection and one death from fecal transplants containing drug-resistant bacteria

	Study	Population	Type of intervention	Results
SDD				
☺	Price et al. [30]	Meta-analysis of 29 articles that enrolled patients in general intensive care units	SDD	Favorable effect on mortality, with a direct evidence odds ratio of 0.73 (95% confidence interval 0.64 to 0.84)
☺	Buelow et al. [31]	10 ICU patients	SDD	The limited risks for antibiotic resistance SDD related
☺	Webster et al. [32]	Meta-analysis of 37 trials (involving more than 7000 patients)	SDD	SDD reduces ventilator-associated pneumonia (odds ratio (OR) = 0.28; 95% confidence interval (CI) = 0.20–0.38) and mortality (OR = 0.73; CI = 0.64–0.84)
Antimicrobial therapy under the control of the metabolic activity of the gut microbiota				
☺	Beloborodova and Sarshor [33]	56 patients with pneumonia or abdominal infection	Enteral correction of the metabolic activity of the gut microbiota	The downward trend of mortality by 11%

Table 1. Generalized data on the possible current use of microbiome therapy.

basis, the use of live bioculture drugs (probiotics) in critically ill patients looks far from harmless and even dangerous. Possible, a NGS-based approach for the detection of bacteremia in patients with sepsis, which has shown promising results, will be a key step in the clinical use of NGS in this indication [35]. In randomized double-blind placebo-controlled independent study on severe acute pancreatitis patients (n = 298)—Probiotics in Pancreatitis Trial (PROPATRIA)—1 group (n = 153), for prophylaxis of suppurative complications received a biomedicine containing 4 species of lactic bacterial (*L. acidophilus, L. casei, L. salivarius, L. lactis*) and 2 species of bifid bacteria (*B. bifidum, B. lactis*) in a dose of 10^{10} daily, while the control group (n = 145) received placebo. The results disappointed the researches: in the group of patients who received probiotics, more severe course of the disease was recorded, necrotizing pancreatitis developed more frequently, secondary bacteremia and other infectious complications occurred, multiple organ failure developed reliably more frequently, and mortality was higher ($p = 0.01$). The authors of the study were unable to provide convincing explanations but expressed their doubts concerning reasonability for use of probiotics in critically ill patients [25].

In our opinion, the use of live microbial cultures of lactic acid bacteria might have aggravated metabolic disturbances and led to adverse consequences in initially severe patients, in particular, because of excessive production of PhLA and p-HPhLA which are typical metabolites of bifido- and lactic bacteria [36, 37]. A group of authors who used probiotics with positive effect in short bowel syndrome patients have reached similar conclusions, namely, the importance of metabolic status evaluation. The colleagues associated high mortality in PROPATRIA study with lethal combination of proteolytic enzymes of pancreas and high level of lactic acid caused by bacterial fermentation of carbohydrates as a key factor related to intake of probiotics. Nevertheless, authors suggest that a probiotic therapy may not be counterindicated for the prevention of secondary infections associated with acute pancreatitis, provided that future clinical studies start probiotic therapy early as possible and prevent bacterial overgrowth not only of patient's own intestinal flora but also the dose of probiotic bacteria [38].

An alternative to probiotics, "smart" direction, is infusion of liquid filtrate of feces from healthy fecal microbiota transplantation. The potential advantage of this method is enlargement of microbial biodiversity and the presence of biologically active substances and metabolites, which might assist a longer effect of microbiota recovery [39]. This procedure has been successfully used for treating the severe infection caused by *Clostridium difficile* in more than 1000 patients [26]. The recent meta-analysis (n = 284) has shown that FMT is significantly more effective in the treatment of such patients compared to the control group in spite of heterogeneity of groups due to the study sites (Europe vs. North America) and method of administration [27]. However, the current experience of FMT application in ICU is limited just to a few patients described only in sporadic publications [28]. The limited quantity of data, absence of objective criteria for efficacy evaluation, and insufficient knowledge of microbiota composition dynamics and its metabolic activity preclude wide application of this method in such vulnerable group of patients. The FDA does not currently approve of any use of fecal transplants. Two patients contracted severe infections, and one of them died, from fecal transplants that contained drug-resistant bacteria [29]. Putting it in another way, given the knowledge and risks, the use of FMT in critically ill patients can be compared to the first blood transfusion before the opening of the ABO system [19].

We assume that the main efforts in fighting infection should be directed to decrease microbial metabolic activity. Considering that the intestine is the main reservoir of bacteria and therefore the main source of bacterial metabolites, it seems appropriate to correct the activity of intestinal microbiota in patient with infection. Enteral correction of the metabolic activity of intestinal microbiota contributes to the improvement of the patients' state [33].

Selective digestive decontamination (SDD) is often considered a prophylactic mode of antibiotic therapy allowing targeted prevention of bowel colonization by "pathogenic" microorganisms. The effect is achieved thanks to the selective impact on potentially pathogenic aerobic and facultative aerobic bacteria by means of enteral administration of antibacterial drugs that do not suppress anaerobic microorganisms, thus creating conditions for recovery of microbiota balance and assisting its functioning even in the unfavorable environment in ICU. Currently, numerous clinical studies and meta-analyses have shown that SDD helps prevent hospital infection in ICU and reduce mortality [30]. Wide implementation of SDD was restricted, inter alia, because of fears of increasing resistance of nosocomial microorganisms to antibiotics [31]; however, convincing data have been obtained confirming the absence of resistant bacterial growth at the background of selective decolonization. A number of major investigations are currently underway, and their authors are expected to give shortly new clinical recommendations concerning the use of this method in ICU [32]. The pronounced clinical effect may be associated with a change in the profile of microbial metabolites, which requires additional research.

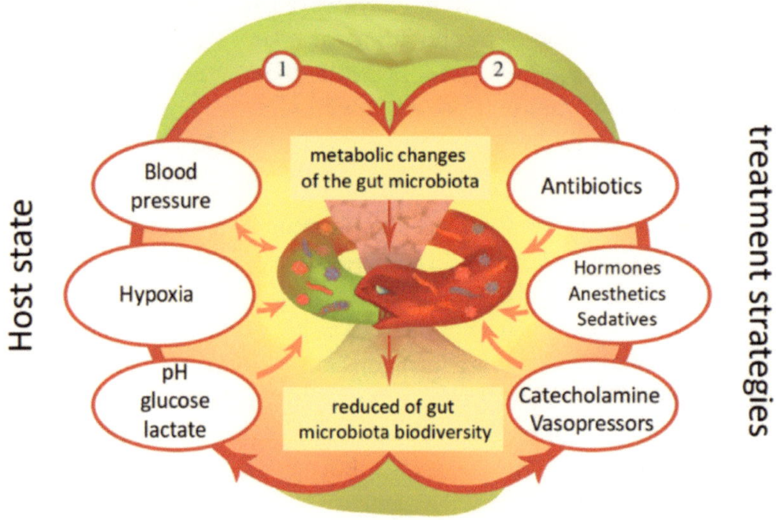

Figure 4. Factors affecting the metabolism of microbiota in ICU [41].

As shown above, the "harmful/beneficial" gut bacteria disbalance is frequently associated with nosocomial pathogens and adverse outcome. The influence of negative factors related to changed internal environment of the macroorganism, and rather aggressive therapy leads to a drastic change in the species diversity of microbiota [40] and, as a consequence, a disturbance of functional activity of microbial community and a development of the maximal disorders that may cause irreversible breakdowns of homeostasis and host body death. A "vicious circle" is created: disturbance of gut microbiome function in critically ill patients leads to overproduction of certain microbial metabolites, which, in turn, have pathological impact on macroorganism's organs and systems (**Figure 4**).

Two potential points of effect in sepsis treatment can be identified as:

1. Host state: prognosing negative dynamics of homeostasis indices as critical condition progresses and maximally sparing regimens of antimicrobial therapy taking into account the important role of microbiome.

2. Treatment strategies: suppression of overgrowth and targeted correction of bacterial metabolism [41].

5. Conclusion

So, are the microbiota-oriented diagnostics and therapy in sepsis a utopia or necessity? In real clinical practice, it is not yet possible to provide real-time monitoring of the microbiome, due to such diagnostics being time-consuming, expensive, complex, and insufficiently studied. Previous works have noted that the gut is a "motor of multiple organ failure and sepsis" [42], and its underestimation earned it a name of "forgotten organ." In the past decades, the number of studies of microbiota in various diseases, including sepsis, has increased drastically and is likely to keep rising. Now it is clear that the "forgotten organ" is a reservoir of pathogens and possibly of genes associated with antibiotic resistance, as well as a marker of disease severity and outcome. Therapy aimed at restoring microbiota equilibrium rather than blindly prescribing broad-spectrum antibiotics may be the best choice. Understanding the metabolic language of microorganisms will serve as a catalyst for the development of new strategies, which will be especially important in the era of antibiotic resistance. New, culturally independent technologies allowing a fast accurate and comprehensive assessment of microbiome will be adapted in the coming years for practical use and wide application. Characterization of changes in ICU patient's microbiome will enable advancement in the development of diagnostic and therapeutic interventions based on changes not only in the microbiota's composition but also in its metabolic profile as well.

6. Methods

We used gas chromatography-mass spectrometry (GC-MS) method to quantify metabolites in human serum from septic patients and healthy volunteers. For taxonomic identification of samples, Ion 16S Metagenomics Kits, Ion Reporter metagenomic workflow solution, and Ion Torrent sequencing systems were used. Clinical and laboratory data and APACHE II and SOFA scores in patients were matched. Data were compared by Mann-Whitney U test; p-values less than 0.05 were considered significant.

Author details

Ekaterina Chernevskaya* and Natalia Beloborodova*

*Address all correspondence to: kate.chernevskaya@gmail.com
and nvbeloborodova@yandex.ru

Federal Research and Clinical Center of Intensive Care Medicine and Rehabilitology, Moscow, Russia

References

[1] Wolff NS, Hugenholtz F, Wiersinga WJ. The emerging role of the microbiota in the ICU. Critical Care. 2018;**22**(1):78. DOI: 10.1186/s13054-018-1999-8

[2] Haak BW, Wiersinga WJ. The role of the gut microbiota in sepsis. The Lancet Gastroenterology and Hepatology. 2017;**2**:135-143. DOI: 10.1016/S2468-1253(16)30119-4

[3] Beloborodova NV, Grechko AV, Olenin AY. Metabolomic discovery of microbiota dysfunction as the cause of pathology. IntechOpen. [Online First] 26 June 2019. DOI:

10.5772/intechopen.87176. Available from: https://www.intechopen.com/online-first/metabolomic-discovery-of-microbiota-dysfunction-as-the-cause-of-pathology

[4] Schmidt K, Mwaigwisya S, Crossman LC, Doumith M, Munroe D, Pires C, et al. Identification of bacterial pathogens and antimicrobial resistance directly from clinical urines by nanopore-based metagenomic sequencing. The Journal of Antimicrobial Chemotherapy. 2017;**72**(1):104-114. DOI: 10.1093/jac/dkw397

[5] Thomas AM, Segata N. Multiple levels of the unknown in microbiome research. BMC Biology. 2019;**17**(1):48. DOI: 10.1186/s12915-019-0667-z

[6] Angus DC, van der Poll T. Severe sepsis and septic shock. The New England Journal of Medicine. 2013;**369**(9):840-851. DOI: 10.1056/NEJMra1208623

[7] Singer M, Deutschman CS, Seymour CW, Shankar-Hari M, Annane D, Bauer M, et al. The third international consensus definitions for sepsis and septic shock (Sepsis-3). Journal of the American Medical Association. 2016;**315**(8):801-810. DOI: 10.1001/jama.2016.0287

[8] Dickson RP. The lung microbiome and ARDS. It is time to broaden the model. American Journal of Respiratory and Critical Care Medicine. 2018;**197**(5):549-551. DOI: 10.1164/rccm.201710-2096ED

[9] Ramsey M, Hartke A, Huycke M. The physiology and metabolism of enterococci. In: Gilmore MS, Clewell DB, Ike Y, Shankar N, editors. Enterococci: From Commensals to Leading Causes of Drug Resistant Infection [Internet]. Boston: Massachusetts Eye and Ear Infirmary; 2014

[10] Weledji EP, Ngowe MN. The challenge of intra-abdominal sepsis. International Journal of Surgery. 2013;**11**(4):290-295. DOI: 10.1016/j.ijsu.2013.02.021

[11] Yeh A, Rogers MB, Firek B, Neal MD, Zuckerbraun BS, Morowitz MJ. Dysbiosis across multiple body sites in critically ill adult surgical patients. Shock. 2016;**46**(6):649-654. DOI: 10.1097/SHK.0000000000000691

[12] Scheiman J, Luber JM, Chavkin TA, MacDonald T, Tung A, Pham LD, et al. Meta-omics analysis of elite athletes identifies a performance-enhancing microbe that functions via lactate metabolism. Nature Medicine. 2019;**25**(7):1104-1109. DOI: 10.1038/s41591-019-0485-4

[13] Beloborodova NV. Chapter 1. Interaction of host-microbial metabolism in sepsis. In: Kumar V editor. Sepsis. Croatia, Rijeka: InTech; 2017. p. 3-19. DOI: 10.5772/68046. Print ISBN 978-953-51-3395-7, 158 pages. DOI: 10.5772/65611. Available from: https://www.intechopen.com/books/sepsis

[14] Jenner AM, Rafter J, Halliwell B. Human fecal water content of phenolics: The extent of colonic exposure to aromatic compounds. Free Radical Biology and Medicine. 2005;**38**(6):763-772. DOI: 10.1016/j.freeradbiomed.2004.11.020

[15] Knarreborg A, Miquel N, Granli T, Jensen BB. Establishment and application of an in vitro methodology to study the effects of organic acids on coliform and lactic acid

bacteria in the proximal part of the gastrointestinal tract of piglets. Animal Feed Science and Technology. 2002;**99**(1):131-140. DOI: 10.1016/S0377-8401(02)00069-X

[16] Beloborodova NV. Sepsis—Metabolomic Approach. Moscow: Meditsin-skoe Informatsionnoe Agentstvo; 2018. 272p. ISBN: 978-5-9986-0350-1. [In Russ.]

[17] Beloborodova NV. Integration of metabolism in man and his microbiome in critical conditions. General Reanimatology. 2012;**8**(4):42-54. DOI: 10.15360/1813-9779-2012-4-42. [In Russ., In Engl.]

[18] Fedotcheva NI, Kazakov RE, Kondrashova MN, Beloborodova NV. Toxic effects of microbial phenolic acids on the functions of mitochondria. Toxicology Letters. 2008;**180**(3):182-188. DOI: 10.1016/j.toxlet.2008.06.861

[19] Chernevskaya E, Beloborodova NV, Bulychev A. Potential contribution of aromatic microbial metabolites to platelet aggregation disturbance. Intensive Care Medicine Experimental. 2018;**6**(Suppl 1):P41. DOI: 10.1186/s40635-018-0196-z

[20] Beloborodova NV, Sarshor YN, Bedova AY, Chernevskaya EA, Pautova AK. Involvement of aromatic metabolites in the pathogenesis of septic shock. Shock. 2018;**50**:273. DOI: 10.1097/shk.0000000000001064

[21] Panigrahi P, Chandel DS, Hansen NI, Sharma N, Kandefer S, Parida S, et al. Neonatal sepsis in rural India: Timing, microbiology and antibiotic resistance in a population-based prospective study in the community setting. Journal of Perinatology. 2017;**37**(8):911-921. DOI: 10.1038/jp.2017.67

[22] Stadlbauer V, Horvath A, Komarova I, Schmerboeck B, Feldbacher N, Klymiuk I, et al. Dysbiosis in early sepsis can be modulated by a multispecies probiotic: A randomised controlled pilot trial. Beneficial Microbes. 2019;**10**(3):265-278. DOI: 10.3920/BM2018.0067

[23] Manzanares W, Lemieux M, Langlois PL, Wischmeyer PE. Probiotic and synbiotic therapy in critical illness: A systematic review and meta-analysis. Critical Care. 2016;**19**:262. DOI: 10.1186/s13054-016-1434-y. PMID:27538711

[24] Kasatpibal N, Whitney JD, Saokaew S, Kengkla K, Heitkemper MM, Apisarnthanarak A. Effectiveness of probiotic, prebiotic, and synbiotic therapies in reducing postoperative complications: A systematic review and network meta-analysis. Clinical Infectious Diseases. 2017;**64**(suppl_2):S153-S160. DOI: 10.1093/cid/cix114

[25] Besselink MG, van Santvoort HC, Buskens E, Boermeester MA, van Goor H, Timmerman HM, et al. Dutch acute pancreatitis study group. Probiotic prophylaxis in predicted severe acute pancreatitis: A randomised, double-blind, placebo-controlled trial. Lancet. 2008;**371**(9613):651-659. DOI: 10.1016/S0140-6736(08)60207-X

[26] Han S, Shannahan S, Pellish R. Fecal microbiota transplant: Treatment options for *Clostridium difficile* infection in the intensive care unit. Journal of Intensive Care Medicine. 2015;**31**(9):577-586. DOI: 10.1177/0885066615594344

[27] Moayyedi P, Yuan Y, Baharith H, Ford AC. Faecal microbiota transplantation for *Clostridium difficile*-associated diarrhoea: A systematic review of randomised controlled trials. The Medical Journal of Australia. 2017;**207**(4):166-172. DOI: 10.5694/mja17.00295

[28] McClave SA, Patel J, Bhutiani N. Should fecal microbial transplantation be used in the ICU? Current Opinion in Critical Care. 2018;**24**(2):105-111. DOI: 10.1097/MCC.0000000000000489

[29] Important Safety Alert Regarding Use of Fecal Microbiota for Transplantation and Risk of Serious Adverse Reactions Due to Transmission of Multi-Drug Resistant Organisms. FDA.GOV. 13 June 2019. Available from: https://www.fda.gov/news-events/fda-brief/fda-brief-fda-warns-about-potential-risk-serious-infections-caused-multi-drug-resistant-organisms

[30] Price R, MacLennan G, Glen J, SuDDICU Collaboration. Selective digestive or oropharyngeal decontamination and topical oropharyngeal chlorhexidine for prevention of death in general intensive care: systematic review and network meta-analysis. BMJ. 2014;**348**:g2197. DOI: 10.1136/bmj.g2197

[31] Buelow E, Bello González TDJ, Fuentes S, de Steenhuijsen Piters WAA, Lahti L, Bayjanov JR, et al. Comparative gut microbiota and resistome profiling of intensive care patients receiving selective digestive tract decontamination and healthy subjects. Microbiome. 2017;**5**(1):88. DOI: 10.1186/s40168-017-0309-z

[32] Webster F, Weijer C, Todd L, Grimshaw JM, Marshall AP, Cook D, et al. The ethics of future trials: Qualitative analysis of physicians' decision making. Trials. 2016;**17**:12. DOI: 10.1186/s13063-015-1137-8

[33] Beloborodova N, Sarshor Y. The first experience of targeted antibiotics for the regulation of the metabolic activity of the gut microbiota (MAGM) in critically ill patients with pneumonia or abdominal infection. Intensive Care Medicine Experimental. 2018;**6**(Suppl 2):0399. DOI: 10.1186/s40635-018-0201-6

[34] Klingensmith NJ, Coopersmith CM. The gut as the motor of multiple organ dysfunction in critical illness. Critical Care Clinics. 2016;**32**(2):203-212. DOI: 10.1016/j.ccc.2015.11.004

[35] Brenner T, Decker SO, Grumaz S, Stevens P, Bruckner T, Schmoch T, et al. Next-generation sequencing diagnostics of bacteremia in sepsis (Next GeneSiS-Trial): Study protocol of a prospective, observational, noninterventional, multicenter, clinical trial. Medicine (Baltimore). 2018;**97**(6):e9868. DOI: 10.1097/MD.0000000000009868

[36] Beloborodova NV, Khodakova AS, Bairamov IT, Olenin AY. Microbial origin of phenylcarboxylic acids in the human body. Biochemistry (Moscow). 2009;**74**(12):1350-1355

[37] Beloborodova NV, Baĭramov IT, Olenin AI, Fedotcheva NI. Exometabolites of some anaerobic microorganisms of human microflora. Biomeditsinskaya Khimiya. 2011;**57**(1): 95-105. Russian

[38] Bongaerts GP, Severijnen RS. A reassessment of the PROPATRIA study and its implications for probiotic therapy. Nature Biotechnology. 2016;**34**(1):55-63. DOI: 10.1038/nbt.3436

[39] van Nood E, Speelman P, Nieuwdorp M, Keller J. Fecal microbiota transplantation: Facts and controversies. Current Opinion in Gastroenterology. 2014;**30**(1):34-39. DOI: 10.1097/MOG.0000000000000024

[40] Dickson RP. The microbiome and critical illness. The Lancet Respiratory Medicine. 2016;**4**(1):59-72. DOI: 10.1016/S2213-2600(15)00427-0

[41] Chernevskaya E, Beloborodova N. Gut microbiome in critical illness (review). General Reanimatology. 2018;**14**:96. DOI: 10.15360/1813-9779-2018-5-96-119

[42] Marshall JC. Gastrointestinal flora and its alterations in critical illness. Current Opinion in Clinical Nutrition and Metabolic Care. 1999;**2**(5):405-411. DOI: 10.1097/00075197-199909000-00009

Chapter 4

Cytokine Gene Polymorphism and Sepsis

Dablu Lal Gupta, Tejparkash Sinha,
Sanjeev Bhoi and D.N. Rao

Additional information is available at the end of the chapter

http://dx.doi.org/10.5772/intechopen.90572

Abstract

Trauma is a significant problem across the globe with mortality more than 50%. Despite the advancement of pre-hospital care to trauma patients, early resuscitation in the emergency department, surgical interventions and intensive care monitoring mortality rate has not improved yet. The higher rate of mortality in trauma patients is usually associated with development of complications such as sepsis, septic shock, and MOF which may occur due to hysterical immune inflammatory responses. Trauma patients who developed these complications in the ICU have comparatively higher chances of mortality. Cytokines are very important for host immune response against infections and play vital roles in the regulation of innate and adaptive immunity. The slanted expression of cytokines due to trauma may be involved in development of sepsis and related complications. The recently published work from various studies suggested that slanted expression of cytokines correlates with the variations in the promoter and structural regions of cytokine genes, which may be responsible for inter-individual differences in susceptibility to sepsis. Therefore, understanding the variations in cytokine genes and associated outcomes due to trauma would possibly contribute to the event of latest genetically changed diagnostic and therapeutic interventions that will improve the outcome in post-traumatic sepsis patients.

Keywords: trauma, cytokine, multiple organ failure, septic shock and inflammation

1. Introduction

Trauma remains a significant public health issue and is the fourth leading cause of death in persons younger than 40 years [1, 2]. Worldwide, about 16,000 people die every day as a result of an injury (5.8 million deaths per year), and the projections for 2020 show that 8.4 million deaths per year are expected [3]. Consequently, injury will be the second most common cause of disability adjusted years of life lost within the next 13 years (second only to cardiovascular disease). Undoubtedly, the major burden of injury is increasingly occurring in the developing world as it industrializes, adopts motorized transportation, and remains the major center for armed conflict [4, 5]. Despite advancement in primary care to trauma patients, early resuscitation in the emergency department, surgical interventions, and intensive care monitoring, mortality rate has not improved yet. The higher rate of mortality to trauma patients is usually associated with development of various complications such as sepsis, septic shock, and the development of the multiple organ dysfunction syndrome (MODS) [6, 7]. The outcome of trauma patients is not determined only by trauma but also by the impacts of immune-inflammatory insult. The inflammatory response is crucial for the host defense against infections, but hysterical immune inflammatory responses are generated due to imbalance in the production of inflammatory and anti-inflammatory cytokines which may lead to various complications and consequently unfavorable outcomes [8, 9]. According to the biphasic model of trauma etiology, dysregulations in the production of both inflammatory and anti-inflammatory cytokines primarily lead to the sepsis-associated mortalities and outcomes [10, 11]. Posttraumatic sepsis which may cause hysterical immune inflammatory responses is one of the leading sources of MODS in the ICU. Although there have been many advances in the development of broad and narrow spectrum of antibiotics and thoughtful care, sepsis remains a serious and deadly problem with high mortality rates across the globe. Therefore, prognostic biomarkers to identify high-risk trauma patients in the early stages are immediately needed for early detection and preventive care of sepsis. The management of severely injured and multiple trauma patients who developed sepsis, septic shock, and MODS due to inflammatory insults is challenging for the physician in the ICU. Trauma leads to imbalance in production of pro-inflammatory and anti-inflammatory cytokines which may subsequently lead to the SIRS, sepsis, septic shock, and MODS which are shown in **Figure 1**.

1.1. SIRS

Systemic inflammatory response syndrome (SIRS) is a term that was developed in an attempt to describe the clinical manifestations that result from the systemic response to injury. The criteria of SIRS are considered as having at least two of the following four clinical parameters abnormal:

1. Temperature < 36°C or > 38° C
2. Heart rate > 90 beats/min
3. Respiratory rate > 20 breaths/min or $Paco_2 < 32$ mm Hg
4. WBC count >12,000 cells/μL or < 4000 cells/μL, or > 10% immature forms

1.2. Sepsis

Sepsis is a common, deadly, and often underappreciated disease process in emergency departments. In the intensive care unit, if patients have SIRS along with documented cultures reports

http://dx.doi.org/10.5772/intechopen.90572

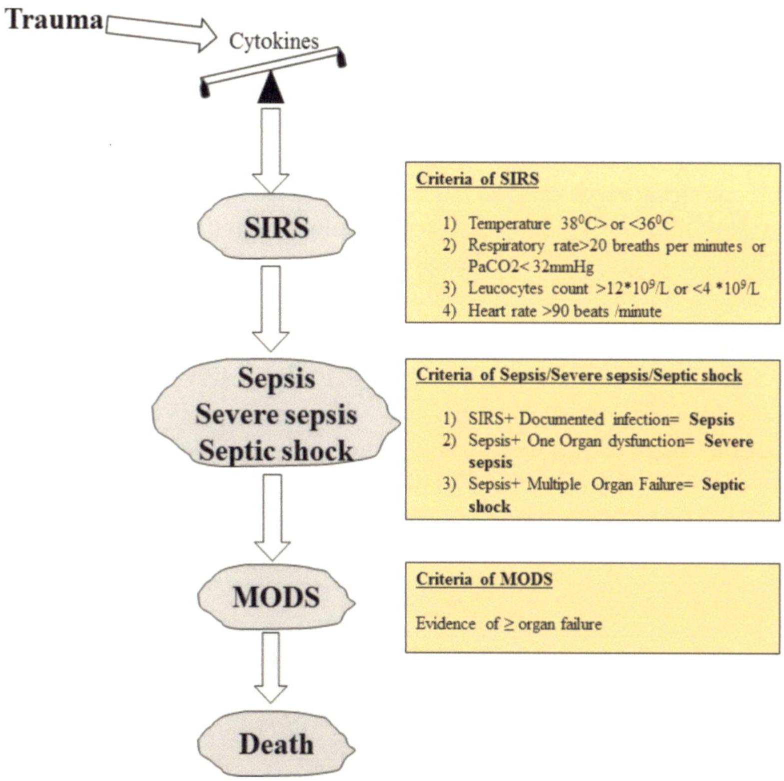

Figure 1. This figure shows that trauma leads to the imbalanced cytokine production which may subsequently lead to the sepsis, severe sepsis, septic shock, MODS, and at last death. This figure also shows the criteria which are used to define the SIRS sepsis, severe sepsis, septic shock, and MODS.

positive is called sepsis. Sepsis results in physiologic alterations that occur at the capillary endothelial level.

1.3. Severe sepsis

Sepsis accompanied by signs of failure of at least one organ. Cardiovascular failure is typically manifested with hypotension, respiratory failure by hypoxemia, renal failure by oliguria, and hematologic failure by coagulopathy.

1.4. Septic shock

Severe sepsis with organ hypoperfusion and hypotension that are poorly responsive to initial fluid resuscitation.

2. Multiple organ failure (MOF)

Multiple organ failure is a clinical syndrome in which the functionality of several organs fails subsequently or simultaneously (i.e., liver, lungs, kidneys, heart). Multiple organ failure after trauma has a multifactorial etiology, which can be divided in endogenous and exogenous factors [12]. The endogenous factors, such as genetic predisposition, form the basis of the patient's susceptibility for the development of organ failure. Recent studies have shown that genetic variations (e.g., TNF-α polymorphisms) are strongly associated with the development of organ failure [13]. The exogenous factors, such as injury itself (the "first hit" or "trauma load") and the resuscitation or surgical intervention (the "second hit" or "intervention load"), play a crucial role in the development of organ failure. Organ damage and subsequent organ failure are the result of dysfunctional immune system [11, 14].

3. Role of cytokines in development of sepsis-related complications

Cytokines are low molecular weight polypeptides, and pharmacologically active molecules possess autocrine, paracrine, and juxtracrine effects [15]. These molecules are classified into several classes (i.e., interleukins, interferons, colony-stimulating factors, tumor necrosis factors,

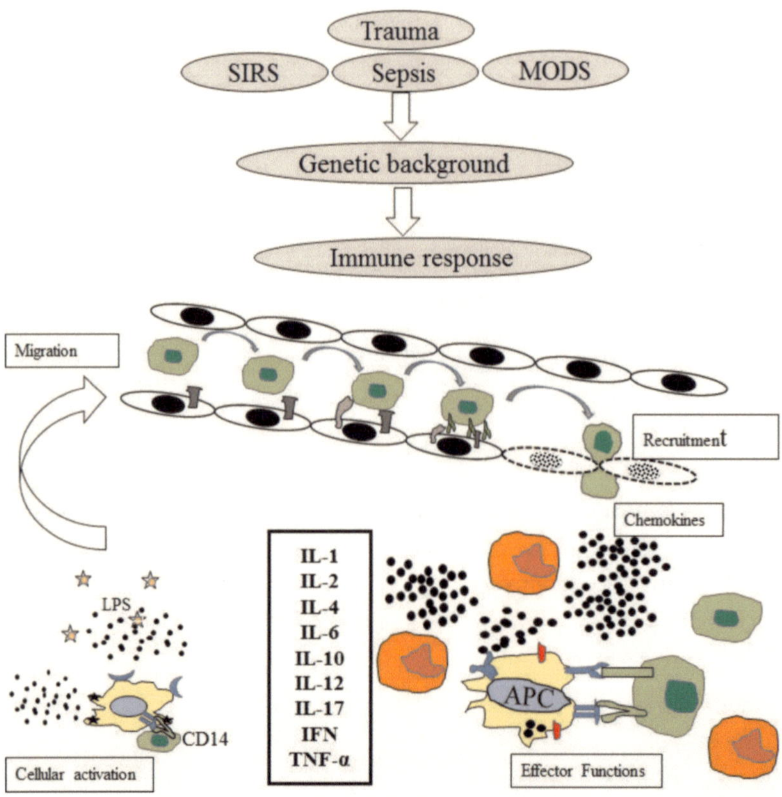

Figure 2. The outcome of trauma patients depends on induced inflammatory response due to trauma such as migration of leukocytes, cellular activation, and effecter functions, which may subsequently depend on genetic background of individuals.

transforming growth factors, and chemokines), which are relevant to mediate the humoral and cellular immunity to protect the host against pathogens [16]. Cytokines are produced by a wide variety of lymphoid and nonlymphoid cells in the body, playing an important role in many physiological responses against infections and injury. In addition, cytokines exert important pleiotropic actions as cardinal effectors of injury [17]. They play vital roles in the regulation of host immune response, and distorted expression of cytokines is proven to be involved in development of complications such as sepsis, septic shock, and MODS. Many studies suggested that the genetic background of individuals determines the impacts of immune inflammatory response after trauma which may lead to differential cellular activations of immune cells, leukocyte migrations, and effector functions (**Figure 2**). Previous research suggests that the variations in the genes encoding cytokines are also involved in the inflammatory responses and also responsible for inter-individual differences in susceptibility to sepsis and in its severity [13, 18, 19]. Therefore, understanding the variations in cytokine genes and associated differences in response to trauma might contribute to the development of new genetically modified diagnostic and therapeutic interventions that may improve outcome in posttraumatic sepsis patients.

4. Role of cytokine gene polymorphism in sepsis

Cytokine gene polymorphism, therefore, is advocated as the underlying reason to distinguish individual specific immune responses. The cytokine gene polymorphism studies may be considered as powerful biomarkers for the identification of trauma patients who have higher risk to develop sepsis complications in the ICU [20, 21]. Therefore, understanding the associations between genetic polymorphisms and sepsis or MODS may lead to the better understanding of sepsis. Nowadays the significance of genetic variations [particularly single-nucleotide polymorphisms (SNPs)] as key determinants of inter-individual variations in both inflammatory responses and clinical outcome in trauma patients is advocated [13, 22]. Single-nucleotide polymorphisms are the key factors to regulate the expressional variation of human genes and found to be associated with the disease susceptibility and progression. To understand the importance of cytokine gene polymorphism (CGP) while predicting the occurrence of sepsis, the SNPs in the promoter, coding, and noncoding regions of 13 cytokine genes with 22 loci are commonly used. Single-nucleotide polymorphisms of 13 cytokine genes including interleukin IL-1-α (T/C-889), IL-1-β (-511 C/T, T/C + 3962), IL-1 RA (T/C mspal 1100), IL-4 RA (G/A + 1902), IL-4(T/G-1098, T/C-590, T/C-33), IL-6 (G/C-174, G/A nt560), IL-10 (G/C-1082, C/T-819, C/A-592), IL-12 (C/A-1188), γIFN (+874 A/T), TGF-β1(C/T codon 10, G/C codon 25), TNF α (G/A -308, G/A-238), and IL-2(T/G-330 G/T + 166), to investigate the susceptibility towards sepsis in trauma patients, are commonly used. All the cytokine genes and their polymorphic loci which are commonly used to investigate the genetic basis of susceptibility towards disease are shown in **Table 1.** Various studies also showed the associations of these SNPs in the development of sepsis and outcomes. The polymorphic loci in the promoter region of TNF-α-308 and TNF-α-238 have been reported by various studies and showed susceptibility and resistance between populations [23, 24]. These two polymorphisms are well recognized and associated with susceptibility for tuberculosis, heart disease, and Graves' disease [25–27]. The interleukin 6 is an important cytokine and plays a very important role in the activation of T17 cells. The polymorphisms in the promoter region of IL-6 (−174 G/C) and structural region (+560) are well characterized in various diseases. However, the polymorphism in the promoter regions (−174G/C) showed significant association with celiac disease, bowel syndrome, cancer, and autoimmunity [28–31]. Interestingly, the polymorphism in the promoter region of IL-6 (−174 G/C) influenced the immunopathogenesis of sepsis and associated with outcomes in European population of trauma [32, 33]. We have also reported the association of IL-6 (−174 G/C) polymorphism and susceptibility of sepsis in the Indian trauma patients [34]. IL-10 is an important anti-inflammatory cytokine and plays a very crucial role in the inflammation, autoimmunity, and tolerance. Many studies suggested that elevated level of IL-10 activates the transcription factor Fox P3 which may subsequently lead to the production T regulatory cells. Polymorphism in the promoter regions of IL-10 gene −1082(G/A), −819(C/T), and − 592 (C/A) is well established and showed significant association with various infectious diseases, autoimmunity, cancer D, and diabetic retinopathy [35–37]. These IL-10 promoters, −1082(G/A), −819(C/T), and − 592(C/A) polymorphisms, are associated with resistance to sepsis in the Caucasian population [38, 39]. Interleukin (IL-1) gene complex consists of IL-1α, IL-1β, IL-1R, and IL-RA genes with five potent polymorphic loci in the structural and promoter regions [40]. These polymorphic loci are associated with susceptibility for sepsis in trauma patients of the Chinese population [41, 42] and also associated with other diseases, such as cancer and autoimmunity [43, 44]. In our study, we have reported the changes in alleles and genotype frequency at the promoter region of IL-1β (−511) gene. We have also reported the significant association of this polymorphism with susceptibility for sepsis in Indian trauma patients. The recently published work by Gupta et al., 2016, showed that polymorphisms in the structural and promoter regions of TNF-α, IL-β, IL-6, and IL-10 are significantly associated with susceptibility to sepsis and outcomes in trauma patients [34] (**Figure 3**).

S.No	Allelic specificity(based on SNP nomenclature commonly used in literature	Corresponding Genotype/Haplotype	Size of the allele-specific amplicon (bp)	Size of the amplication control (bp) CRPgene-90bp/β-globin gene-440bp	Name of the cytokine
1	T at pos. -889	T	220bp	440bp	IL-1α
2	Cat pos.-889	C	220bp	440bp	IL-1α
3	C at pos.-511	C	215bp	440bp	IL-1β
4	T at pos. -511	T	215bp	440bp	IL-1β
5	T at pos.+3962	T	340bp	440bp	IL-1β
6	C at pos.+3962	C	340bp	440bp	IL-1β
7	C at pos.pstl 1970	C	290bp	440bp	IL-1R
8	T at pos.pstl 1970	T	290bp	440bp	IL-1R
9	T at pos.mspall11100	T	300bp	440bp	IL-1RA
10	C at pos.mspall11100	C	300bp	440bp	IL-1RA
11	G at pos.+1902	G	140bp	440bp	IL-4R
12	A at pos.+1902	A	140bp	440bp	IL-4R
13	C at pos.-1188	C	800bp	440bp	IL-12
14	A at pos-1188bp	A	800bp	440bp	IL-12
15	A at pos.+874	A	180bp	440bp	IFN-Y
16	T at pos.+874	T	180bp	440bp	IFN-Y
17	C at codon 10;G at codon 25	CG	80bp	440bp	TGF-β
18	C at codon 10;C at codon 25	CC	80bp	440bp	TGF-β
19	T at codon 10;G at codon 25	TG	80bp	440bp	TGF-β
20	T at codon 10;C at codon 25	TC	80bp	440bp	TGF-β

21	C at codon 10	CG or CC	195bp	440bp	TGF-β
22	C at codon 10	TG or TC	195bp	440bp	TGF-β
23	G at pos.-308;G at pos.-238	GG	110bp	440bp	TNF-α
24	G at pos.-308;G at pos.-238	AG	110bp	440bp	TNF-α
25	G at pos.-308;G at pos.-238	GA	110bp	440bp	TNF-α
26	A at pos.-308;A at pos.-238	AA	110bp	440bp	TNF-α
27	T at pos.-330bp;G at pos.-238	TG	560bp	440bp	IL-2
28	G at pos.-330bp;G at pos.-238	GG	560bp	440bp	IL-2
29	G at pos.-330bp;G at pos.-238	GT	560bp	440bp	IL-2
30	T at pos.-330bp;T at pos.-238	TT	560bp	440bp	IL-2
31	T at pos.-10-98;T at pos-590	TT	560bp	90bp	IL-4
32	T at pos.-10-98;C at pos-590	TC	560bp	90bp	IL-4
33	G at pos.-10-98;T at pos-590	GT	560bp	90bp	IL-4
34	G at pos.-10-98;C at pos-590	GC	560bp	90bp	IL-4
35	T at pos.-590;T at pos-33	TT	560bp	90bp	IL-4
36	T at pos.-590;TCat pos-33	TC	610bp	90bp	IL-4
37	C at pos.-590;T at pos-33	CT	610bp	90bp	IL-4
38	C at pos.-590;C at pos-33	CC	610bp	90bp	IL-4
39	G at pos-174;G at pos+565	GG	610bp	90bp	IL-6
40	C at pos-174;G at pos+565	CG	430bp	90bp	IL-6
41	G at pos-174;A at pos+565	GA	430bp	90bp	IL-6
42	C at pos-174;A at pos+565	CA	430bp	90bp	IL-6
43	G at pos-1082;C at pos-819	GC*=GCC or GCA	430bp	90bp	IL-10
44	G at pos-1082;C at pos-592	G*C=GCC or GAC	305bp	90bp	IL-10
45	A at pos-1082;C at pos-819	AC*=ACC or ACA	305bp	90bp	IL-10
46	A at pos-1082;T at pos-819	AT*=ATC or ATA	305bp	90bp	IL-10
47	A at pos-1082;C at pos-592	A*C=ACC o ATC	305bp	90bp	IL-10
48	A at pos-1082;A at pos-592	A*A=ACA or ATA	530bp	90bp	IL-10

Table 1. Twenty-two single-nucleotide polymorphism in 13 cytokine genes including structural and coding regions.

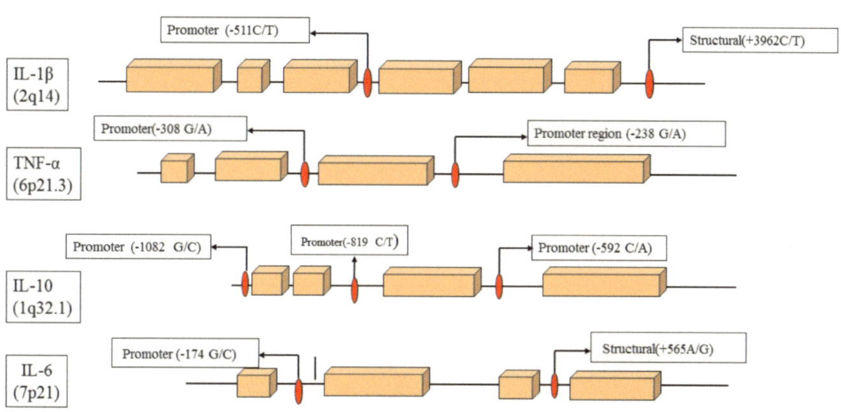

Figure 3. This figure shows the cytokine genes and its polymorphic loci present in the structural and promoter regions which are significantly involved in susceptibility for sepsis, septic shock, and death.

5. Conclusion

The purpose of this chapter is to bring together currently available information of cytokine gene polymorphisms in pro-inflammatory and anti-inflammatory cytokine genes in the development of various complications such as sepsis, septic shock, and MODS in trauma patients. Specific emphasis is placed on the polymorphism of those cytokines which potentially contributed to the development of these complications and correlates with unfavorable outcomes.

Acknowledgements

This work was funded through the Indian Council of Medical Research (ICMR), New Delhi. The author is thankful to the University Grant Commission (UGC), New Delhi, India, for fellowship assistance. The excellent scientific assistance of Dr. Vinay, Dr. Amit Gupta, and Dr. Arul Selvi is acknowledged.

Conflict of interest

The authors have no conflicts of interest.

Author details

Dablu Lal Gupta[1]*, Tejparkash Sinha[2], Sanjeev Bhoi[2] and D.N. Rao[3]

*Address all correspondence to: dablugupta10@gmail.com

1 Institute of Science, Nirma University, Ahmedabad, Gujarat, India

2 Department of Emergency Medicine, JPN Apex Trauma Center, All India Institute of Medical Sciences, New Delhi, India

3 Department of Biochemistry, All India Institute of Medical Science, New Delhi, India

References

[1] Rittirsch D, Flierl MA, Ward PA. Harmful molecular mechanisms in sepsis. Nature Reviews. Immunology. Oct. 2008;**8**(10):776-787

[2] Moore K. Trauma mortality: Understanding mortality distribution to improve outcomes. Journal of Emergency Nursing. Jul. 2014;**40**(4):405-406

[3] Mikkelsen R, Møller Hansen O, Brink O. Non-survivors after admission to trauma Centre. Danish Medical Journal. Oct. 2014;**61**(10):A4928

[4] Spence RT, Scott JW, Haider A, Navsaria PH, Nicol AJ. Comparative assessment of in-hospital trauma mortality at a South African trauma center and matched patients treated in the United States. Surgery. 2017;**162**(3):620-627

[5] Luu MH, Cramer CL, Cabezas MN, Soshnik-Schierling L, Barnhardt WF, Young JS. The evolution of trauma care: Relative mortality analysis at a level 1 trauma center over two decades. The American Surgeon. Aug. 2017;**83**(8):e274-e276

[6] Nguyen HB et al. Severe sepsis and septic shock: Review of the literature and emergency department management guidelines. Annals of Emergency Medicine. Jul. 2006;**48**(1):54.e1

[7] Bone RC, Grodzin CJ, Balk RA. Sepsis: A new hypothesis for pathogenesis of the disease process. Chest. Jul. 1997;**112**(1):235-243

[8] Gupta DL, Bhoi S, Mohan T, Galwnkar S, Rao DN. Coexistence of Th1/Th2 and Th17/Treg imbalances in patients with post traumatic sepsis. Cytokine. 2016;**88**:214-221

[9] Cecconi M, Evans L, Levy M, Rhodes A. Sepsis and septic shock. Lancet. Jul. 2018; **392**(10141):75-87

[10] Chakraborty S, Karasu E, Huber-Lang M. Complement after trauma: Suturing innate and adaptive immunity. Frontiers in Immunology. 2018;**9**:2050

[11] Hietbrink F, Koenderman L, Rijkers G, Leenen L. Trauma: The role of the innate immune system. World Journal of Emergency Surgery: WJES. May 2006;**1**:15

[12] Ramírez M. Multiple organ dysfunction syndrome. Current Problems in Pediatric and Adolescent Health Care. Dec. 2013;**43**(10):273-277

[13] Majetschak M et al. Relation of a TNF gene polymorphism to severe sepsis in trauma patients. Annals of Surgery. Aug. 1999;**230**(2):207

[14] Cohen J. The immunopathogenesis of sepsis. Nature. Dec. 2002;**420**(6917):885-891

[15] Lanas A, Sekar MC, Hirschowitz BI. Objective evidence of aspirin use in both ulcer and nonulcer upper and lower gastrointestinal bleeding. Gastroenterology. Sep. 1992;**103**(3): 862-869

[16] Yao YM, Luan Y. Precision evaluation of immune status and its significance in sepsis after burns or trauma. Zhonghua Shao Shang Za Zhi. Nov. 2018;**34**(11):786-789

[17] Chang HR, Bistrian B. The role of cytokines in the catabolic consequences of infection and injury. JPEN Journal of Parenteral and Enteral Nutrition. Jun. 1998;**22**(3):156-166

[18] Zhao Y et al. The -144C/A polymorphism in the promoter of HSP90beta is associated with multiple organ dysfunction scores. PLoS One. Mar. 2013;**8**(3):e58646

[19] Fowler EV. TNF and IL10 SNPs act together to predict disease behaviour in Crohn's disease. Journal of Medical Genetics. Jun. 2005;**42**(6):523-528

[20] Stanilova SA, Miteva LD, Stanilov NS, Stefanov CS, Karakolev ZT. Interleukin-12b polymorphisms in association with susceptibility to severe sepsis. Laboratoriums Medizin. Jan. 2010;**41**(1):47-50

[21] Bauer I et al. Influence of gender on stimulated cytokine response in patients with severe sepsis. Anaesthesist. May 2006;**55**(5):515-527

[22] Bidwell J et al. Cytokine gene polymorphism in human disease: On-line databases. Genes and Immunity. Sep. 1999;**1**(1):3-19

[23] Gordon AC et al. TNF and TNFR polymorphisms in severe sepsis and septic shock: A prospective multicentre study. Genes and Immunity. Dec. 2004;**5**(8):631-640

[24] Azevedo ZM et al. Tumor necrosis factor (TNF) and lymphotoxin-alpha (LTA) single nucleotide polymorphisms: Importance in ARDS in septic pediatric critically ill patients. Human Immunology. Jun. 2012;**73**(6):661-667

[25] Ceylan E, Karkucak M, Coban H, Karadag M, Yakut T. Evaluation of TNF-alpha gene (G308A) and MBL2 gene codon 54 polymorphisms in Turkish patients with tuberculosis. Journal of Infection and Public Health. Dec. 2017;**10**(6):774-777

[26] Huangfu F, Zhao X, Wang X, Tang L, Jiang J. There is no association between TNF-α gene polymorphisms and the risk of coronary artery heart disease: A meta-analysis. The Journal of Cardiovascular Surgery. Oct. 2017;**58**(5):770-778

[27] Tu Y, Fan G, Zeng T, Cai X, Kong W. Association of TNF-α promoter polymorphism and Graves' disease: An updated systematic review and meta-analysis. Bioscience Reports. 2018;**38**(2):27

[28] Akbulut UE, Çebi AH, Sağ E, İkbal M, Çakır M. Interleukin-6 and interleukin-17 gene polymorphism association with celiac disease in children. The Turkish Journal of Gastroenterology. Nov. 2017;**28**(6):471-475

[29] Bashashati M, Moradi M, Sarosiek I. Interleukin-6 in irritable bowel syndrome: A systematic review and meta-analysis of IL-6 (-G174C) and circulating IL-6 levels. Cytokine. 2017; **99**:132-138

[30] Zhai K, Yang Y, Gao Z-G, Ding J. Interleukin-6-174G>C gene promoter polymorphism and prognosis in patients with cancer. Oncotarget. Jul. 2017;**8**(27):44490-44497

[31] Hu S et al. Association between IL-6-174G/C polymorphism and risk of multiple sclerosis: A meta-analysis. Genetic Testing and Molecular Biomarkers. Feb. 2014;**18**(2):127-130

[32] Jeremić V et al. Clinical relevance of IL-6 gene polymorphism in severely injured patients. Bosnian Journal of Basic Medical Sciences. 2014;**14**(2):110-117

[33] Sapan HB et al. Pattern of cytokine (IL-6 and IL-10) level as inflammation and anti-inflammation mediator of multiple organ dysfunction syndrome (MODS) in polytrauma. International Journal of Burns and Trauma. 2016;**6**(2):37-43

[34] Gupta DL, Nagar PK, Kamal VK, Bhoi S, Rao DN. Clinical relevance of single nucleotide polymorphisms within the 13 cytokine genes in north Indian trauma hemorrhagic shock patients. Scandinavian Journal of Trauma, Resuscitation and Emergency Medicine. Nov. 2015;**23**:96

[35] Wu H, Guo J, He Y, Yin H, Shu J. Relationship between IL-10 gene -819C/T polymorphism and the risk of inflammatory bowel disease: A meta-analysis. African Health Sciences. Sep. 2016;**16**(3):866-872

[36] Sharma N, Toor D. Interleukin-10: Role in increasing susceptibility and pathogenesis of rheumatic fever/rheumatic heart disease. Cytokine. 2017;**90**:169-176

[37] Wattanathum A, Manocha S, Groshaus H, Russell JA, Walley KR. Interleukin-10 haplotype associated with increased mortality in critically ill patients with sepsis from pneumonia but not in patients with extrapulmonary sepsis. Chest. Sep. 2005;**128**(3):1690-1698

[38] Jeremić V, Alempijević T, Mijatović S, Arsenijević V, Ladjevic N, Krstić S. Clinical relevance of IL-10 gene polymorphism in patients with major trauma. Medicinski glasnik (Zenica). Aug. 2014;**11**(2):326-332

[39] Liese AM, Siddiqi MQ, Siegel JH, Deitch EA, Spolarics Z. Attenuated monocyte IL-10 production in glucose-6-phosphate dehydrogenase-deficient trauma patients. Shock. Jul. 2002;**18**(1):18-23

[40] Garlanda C, Dinarello CA, Mantovani A. The interleukin-1 family: Back to the future. Immunity. Dec. 2013;**39**(6):1003-1018

[41] Zhang A-Q et al. Associations between interleukin-1 gene polymorphisms and sepsis risk: A meta-analysis. BMC Medical Genetics. Jan. 2014;**15**:8

[42] Wen A-Q et al. Clinical relevance of IL-1β promoter polymorphisms (−1470, −511, and −31) IN patients with major trauma. Shock. Jun. 2010;**33**(6):576-582

[43] Raza Y et al. Combination of interleukin 1 polymorphism and *Helicobacter pylori* infection: An increased risk of gastric cancer in Pakistani population. Pathology Oncology Research. Oct. 2017;**23**(4):873-880

[44] Fontanella M et al. Interleukin-1 cluster gene polymorphisms and aneurysmal subarachnoid hemorrhage. Neurosurgery. Jun. 2010;**66**(6):1058-1063

Chapter 5

Hemostatic Aspect of Sepsis

Bashir Abdrhman Bashir Mohammed

Additional information is available at the end of the chapter

http://dx.doi.org/10.5772/intechopen.90800

Abstract

The hemostatic system is composed of primary hemostasis and coagulation on the one hand, and natural regulatory anticoagulant protein mechanisms and fibrinolysis, on the other hand. Under physiological conditions, these processes are balanced. Under septic conditions, coagulopathy may followed by disseminated intravascular coagulation (DIC). Tissue factor (TF) pathway is regarded to be the core way for activation of the coagulation cascade in sepsis. TF is triggered by pro-inflammatory mediators, encompassing cytokines, C-reactive protein, and advanced glycation end products in peripheral blood cells and on microparticle molecules. Once a septic patient develops DIC, a significant increase in the susceptibility of developing organ dysfunction, morbidity, and mortality may occur. This work was basic elucidation of the idea that coagulation and its inhibitors are of major importance in coagulation-inflammation noise, similarly as in cure from sepsis.

Keywords: coagulopathy, diagnostic criteria, inflammation, DIC, infection, sepsis

1. Introduction

Sepsis is a confounding clinical condition that emerges when a patient responds unfavorably to a disease and creates organ dysfunction as an outcome. It can influences all the intents and purposes of organ framework; however, organ involvement and the level of dysfunction will change remarkably between patients. It will end in death in extreme cases. Sepsis is these days formally distinct as a dysregulated host reflection to disease, triggering perilous organ pathology [1]. This new definition, working with clinical measures, will ideally give a lot of grounded, increasingly predictable base to better illuminate occurrence, results, and survey. The impact of sepsis is implausibly florid, and therefore the infectious track will vary significantly among patients. So far, sepsis has not been resolved and determined crucially in several cases.

Determination often depends upon the practician pattern as authoritative microbiological proof of Associate in Nursing encouraging contamination is frequently missing. Besides, endeavors to find an association in nursing enchantment remedy and sepsis have been in vain [2].

Management is primarily supported with resuscitation, organ backup and wipe out the dependent contagion with antibiotics ± supply control [2]. On an increasingly affirmative note, our comprehension of sepsis has significantly amplified, and superior diagnostics are being created to help recognizable proof and focus on the potion and timing of restorative medications. In developing nations, sepsis has a consolidated recurrence of 2.5 million patients for each year and demise extent of roughly 650,000 patients consistently [3]. This would mean, usually 19 million instances of sepsis a year, internationally, with roughly 5 million deaths [3]. This estimation is probably going to be uncontrollably inaccurate, as there is a general absence of intensive medical specialty data on low- and middle-income countries. The absence of good essential consideration, sufficient infection control, convenient anti-microbial treatment, poor staffing levels, and satisfactory basic care arrangement represents a totally distinctive circumstance in these nations. The World Health Organization gives extra insight regarding this problem. As indicated by WHO data, three irresistible infections were among the 10 most important reasons for death worldwide in 2015: lower respiratory disorder, diarrheal disease, and tuberculosis with a consolidated mortality of 7.3 million individuals [4].

Most of those fatalities happen in developing countries. Similarly, most die from sepsis as infection, while not organ dysfunction cannot be touch-and-go. The death rate of sepsis is declining within the developing countries, to some extent due to the very fact that of previous acknowledgment and clinical administration nevertheless additionally on the grounds that expanded acknowledgment has considerably expanded the denominator [5]. Sepsis might not usually be recorded because the reason for death may be attributed of various comorbidities, as an example, cancer or cardiovascular issues. Death in a septic patient may be connected to a secondary or an unrelated sequel [6].

2. Sepsis and coagulation

Sepsis is associated with intense and conceivably dangerous sequel of infection. Sepsis happens when host defense mediators are discharged into the circulation to battle the infection evoking fundamental inflammatory responses all through the body [1]. About two-hundredth of patients with infection die within the emergency clinic, and extreme sepsis prompts a death rate of around four-hundredth [3, 4].

Sepsis is reliably connected with coagulation variations [5]. These variations emerge from activation of coagulation that must be distinguished by profoundly delicate examines for hemostatic factor assays to some degree progressively extreme coagulation activation that might be recognizable by an inconspicuous fall in thrombocyte count check and subclinical prolongation of worldwide hemostatic factors characteristics to squeaky disseminated intravascular coagulation (DIC), demonstrated by plentiful microvascular occlusion in very little and medium-size veins and synchronous diffused bleeding from totally different sites [5–7].

Septic patients and intensive cases of DIC might evidence thromboembolic involvements or clinically less clear microvascular clot development, which will boost multiple organ failure [6, 8]. In several cases, intensive hemorrhage may well be the predominant presentation [9]; also, a lot of the time, sepsis and a DIC cause synchronous thrombosis and bleeding. Hemorrhage is owed to consumption and consequent depletion of coagulation factors and platelets, brought by progressing activation of the hemostatic system [10]. Furthermore, this conjunction might present because the Waterhouse-Friderichsen syndrome, unremarkably highlighted throughout fulminant meningococcal septicemia, and despite numerous different microorganisms may cause this clinical circumstance [11].

3. Recurrence of clinically relevant coagulopathy in sepsis

Clinically vital hemostatic changes might happen in up to 70% of septic patients. Furthermore, concerning 35% of patients with sepsis can fulfill the standard criteria for DIC [12, 13]. Most septic patients can create thrombocytopenia (platelet count less than $150 \times 10^9/l$) [14, 15]. Usually, blood thrombocyte count reduces within the initial 4 days following admission to the emergency clinic [16]. The seriousness of sepsis relates uniquely to the decline in platelet count [17]. Basic causes of thrombocytopenia in sepsis are diminished platelet production, upgraded consumption, or sequestration in the spleen. Diminished generation of megakaryocytes in the bone marrow may appear to be indiscernible with the elevated levels of platelet production-stimulating pro-inflammatory mediators, for instance, tumor necrosis factor (TNF)-α and interleukin (IL)-6, and raised values of thrombopoietin in patients with sepsis, which presumptively ought to trigger megakaryopoiesis [18]. However, in a very sizable proportion of septic patients, hemophagocytosis happens, involving dynamic phagocytosis of thrombocyte progenitors and other diverse hematopoietic cells by mononuclear cells, clearly fetching by raising the concentration of macrophage stimulating factor (M-CSF) in sepsis [19]. Thrombocyte utilization is outwardly likewise critical in sepsis, due to thrombocyte activation optional to ongoing advancement of thrombin.

Platelet activation, excessive utilization, and devastation occur at the endothelial surface because of the rule of endothelial cell-platelet interplay in sepsis, even though the degree may differ between completely different vascular beds of assorted organs [20]. Elongation time of hemostatic analyses, like prothrombin clotting time (PT) or the kaolin-cephalin clotting time (KCCT), is noticeable in 15–30% of septic patients [21]. Hemostatic changes involve high fibrin split products items (in quite 95% of patients) [22, 23] and scanty values of natural regulatory anticoagulant proteins, for instance, anti-thrombin and protein C (90% of septic patients) [23, 24].

4. Tracks prompting coagulation adjustments in sepsis

In the recent three decades, the tracks engaged in hemostatic disorder of sepsis are explained for a significant part [7]. Unmistakably different components in the coagulation system act at the same time toward a prohemostatic state. Obviously the most significant variables that intercede with this derangement of the coagulation system during sepsis are cytokines. Abundant proof shows a broad crosstalk among inflammation and coagulation, where alongside inflammation-induced prompted coagulation activation, and coagulation likewise especially impacted inflammatory activity. Notably, comprehensive hemostatic activation and inflammation in sepsis may show with organ-specific observations that are applicable for the particular organ failure ensuing from serious sepsis [25]. The most vital instigator of thrombin generation in sepsis is the transmembrane tissue factor. Investigations of endotoxemia or cytokinemia have exhibited a focal job of the TF/FVIIa combination within the inception of thrombin generation [26]. Repeal of the TF/factor VII (a) pathway by appointed mediations at TF or FVIIa activity realized a total repeal of thrombin generation in experimental scopes [27, 28]. To boot, in serious gram-negative sepsis, ex vivo transmembrane tissue factor expression on monocytes of patients was exhibited [29]. This supported the appraisal of movement of TF from mononuclear cells to activated thrombocytes in associate degree ex vivo insertion setup, it completely was anticipated that this "bloodborne" TF shifts between cells via microparticles [30].

Thrombocytes have a focal activity within the progression of hemostatic variations in sepsis. Thrombocytes could activate straightforwardly by pro-inflammatory cytokine mediators, such as platelet-activating factor [31]. The produced thrombin can then potentiate platelets. Activation of blood platelets might likewise elicit fibrin makeup by elective mechanism. The manifestation of P-selectin on the thrombocyte surface membrane does not simply intervene in the adherence of thrombocytes to leukocytes and endothelial cells; it additionally promotes the aspect of TF on monocytes [32]. In typical conditions, activation of coagulation is controlled by three significant physiological, medicinal, anticoagulant pathways: the antithrombin, the activated protein C, and the tissue factor pathway inhibitor (TFPI). In sepsis, each of the three pathways is considerably affected [33]. Owing to a combination of reduced synthesis, continuous utilization, and proteolytic degradation (e.g., by neutrophil elastase), the levels of each of the three coagulation inhibitors are low. Additionally, noteworthy downregulation of thrombomodulin and endothelial protein C receptor (EPCR) in inflammatory conditions will create an impair diversion of protein C (autoprothrombin IIA) and activated protein C. Eventually, at the time of the massive activation of hemostasis in sepsis, endogenous fibrinolysis is commonly crushed. Afterward, during the acute release of plasminogen activators (tissue-plasminogen activator (t-PA)) and urokinase-plasminogen activator (u-PA) from capacity destinations in vascular endothelial cell structure throughout inflammatory conditions, the augmentation in plasminogen activation and subsequent placement subject production is worked by a upheld increase in plasminogen activator inhibitor-1 (PAI-1) [34]. Apparently, researchers have indicated that a purposeful transformation within the PAI-1 sequence, the 4G/5G polymorphism, not simply influenced the level of PAI-1; but, this was in addition connected to the clinical consequences of gram-negative bacterial sepsis. Patients with the 4G/4G genotype had basically higher PAI-1 levels associated with nursing and distended mortality [35]. Completely different studies indicated that the PAI-1 polymorphism distended the risk of making septic shock from meningococcal contamination [36].

5. Endothelial activation and its impact on coagulation throughout inflammation

Vascular endothelial lining assume a central role altogether element that result in inflammation-induced activation of coagulation. Throughout severe infection, the endothelium is vitalized by pathogens or indirectly through inflammatory mediators and therefore the major restrictive antithrombotic properties become inactivated [25, 37]. Pro-inflammatory cytokines containing interleukin-1 (IL-1), tumor necrosis factor-α (TNF-α), and IL-6 trigger TF inside endothelial cells, which might be shed to some extent as soluble TF [38]. Shedding of soluble TF could clarify why it has been onerous to distinguish endothelial TF by assay in animal studies [39]. It remains questionable whether or not endothelial cells contribute to TF production in sepsis. Taking out the TF gene selectively in endothelial cells did not constrict the level of activated coagulation estimated as a thrombin-ATIII complex when mice were tested with lipopolysaccharide (LPS) [40]. The equivalent pro-inflammatory cytokines seem to downregulate the anticoagulant receptors thrombomodulin (TM) and EPCR, furthermore cellular glycosaminoglycans [41].

Endothelial cells are likewise able to release adhesion particles and growth factors that will not simply advance the inflammatory response nonetheless to boot increment the coagulation response. Combining between platelets and endothelial cells, likewise as platelets and neutrophils, is considerably connected to the beginning of inflammation. In endothelial cells, the Weibel-Palade body secretes von Willebrand factor (VWF) and P-selectin, that backup thrombocyte rolling. Inflamed endothelium bolsters blood leukocyte rolling, and activated platelets in reality with leukocytes. Furthermore, endothelial cells discharge various mediators of the inflammatory response [42]. Such a mediator incorporates CD40 ligand, lipoxygenases, prostaglandins, etc. Of potential pro-coagulant significance are microparticles that are discharged on activation and apoptosis of cells and that arise from virtually any blood cell [43]. Microparticles have indicated procoagulant activity via activation of TF or totally different chemicals in varied disease states, together with meningococcal sepsis [13]. Microparticles have been shown to have a few other biological properties that improve the cardiovascular system. In sepsis, microparticles manage unique inflammatory responses in an organ-specific manner and may assume a job in the appropriation of proteins like APC [44].

6. Inflammation and hemostatic disorders in sepsis

Like essentially all fundamental inflammation impacts of infection, the disturbance of the hemostatic protocol in sepsis is coordinated by many cytokines. Most star pro-inflammatory cytokines are shown to start out the hemostatic activation in vitro. In sepsis, elevated rates of cytokines are often found within the circulation of septic patients and analyses illness or checking endotoxemia may lead to a transient increment in plasma cytokines levels [26]. Tumor necrosis factor (TNF) is the main acolyte that gets discovered, pursued by a rise in serum levels of some interleukins (IL), of which IL-6 and IL-1 are conspicuous. Meanwhile, anti-inflammatory plasma cytokines (like IL-10) may have a brake job in the invigoration of coagulation. As TNF is the essential cytokine to become perceptible in the blood circulation onto bacteremia and this cytokine has powerful procoagulant impacts, it was first thought that hemostatic activation in sepsis was intervened by TNF. However, in a very few preliminary trials numerous procedures to inhibit TNF action, it was demonstrated that endotoxin exhortation of TNF cytokine may be altogether repealed, though activation of blood coagulation was not influenced, nonetheless that the impacts on blood coagulation inhibitors and fibrinolysis perceived to be controlled by TNF cytokine [26]. Strangely, it was exhibited in consequent investigations that techniques that block IL-6 cause a total inhibition of endotoxin-induced activation of coagulation [45]. Additionally, surveys in malignant patients treated with recombinant IL-6 indicated that following the infusion of this cytokine, noticeable thrombin generation happened [46]. Subsequently, these outcomes propose that IL-6 as opposed to TNF cytokine is critical as an inducer for cytokine-triggered blood hemostatic activation. Although IL-1 is associated in nursing intense agonist of TF expression in vitro, its role has not been utterly explained in vivo. An IL-1 receptor adversary principally hindered the procoagulant response in trial sepsis ideals and paused thrombin generation in patients [47]. Moreover, the greater part of the modifications in hemostasis happen well prior to IL-1 getting detected in the blood circulation, leaving a potential function of IL-1 in the coagulopathy of sepsis an agitated issue. Blood coagulation factors and anticoagulant regulatory proteins do not just assume a role in hemostatic activation; they additionally communicate with specific cell receptors prompting the activation of signaling pathways. Particularly, protease interplays that regulate inflammatory operations may well be significant in sepsis. The vital pathway whereby coagulation compartments manage inflammation is by official to protease-activated receptors (PARs). PARs are transmembrane G-protein-coupled receptors; moreover, four distinct sets (PAR 1–4) have been perceived [48]. A typical aspect of PARs is that they fill in as their own ligand. Proteolytic spilt by an activated blood coagulation factor prompts exposure to a neo-amino terminus that is able to activate a same receptor (and likely boarded receptors), prompting transmembrane signaling. PAR-1, PAR-3, and PAR-4 are receptors that are activated by thrombin, whereas PAR-2 is activated by the TF/FVIIa complex, factor Xa, and trypsin enzyme. PAR-1 is in addition a receptor for the TF/FVIIa complex in conjunction with factor Xa. It has become obvious that there is a major crosstalk between blood coagulation inhibitors and inflammatory arbiters additionally. Antithrombin III can render as an organizer of inflammation, for example, by direct link to inflammatory cells, during this approach diminishing cytokine and chemokine receptor manifestation [49]. Likewise, there is plenty of proof that the protein C (PC) order critically regulates inflammatory action [50]. APC has been manifested to constrict endotoxin-induced production of TNF-α, IL-1β, IL-6, and IL-8 cytokines by monocytes/macrophages [51]. APC additionally prevents cytokine discharge and blood leukocyte activation in experimental bacteremia in vivo [52]. The hindrance of the PC shunt by a monoclonal antibody exasperates the inflammatory response, as appeared by promoting levels of pro-inflammatory cytokines and dilated blood leukocyte activation and tissue injury [53]. Mice with a various PC inadequacy due to focused disturbance of the PC gene have not just a vigorous hemostatic response to experimental endotoxemia but conjointly display high contrasts in inflammatory responses (e.g., excess value of plasma pro-inflammatory cytokines) (**Table 1**) [54].

Pro-inflammatory
Interleukin 1β
Interleukin 6
Interleukin 8
Tumor necrosis factor (TNF-α)
Transforming growth factor (TGF-β)
Anti-inflammatory
Interleukin 1 receptor antagonist
IL-4
IL-6
IL-10
IL-11
IL-13
Soluble TNF receptors

Table 1. Some pro-inflammatory and anti-inflammatory cytokines.

7. Role of neutrophil in coagulation in sepsis

In sepsis, the early cytokine storm shows up at intervals of 30–90 minutes during lipopolysaccharide (LPS) layer exposure. The following stage comprises the activation of neutrophils and nitrous oxide, further cytokine discharge, and the formation of kinins, complement protein products, lipid mediators [55, 56], and the tissue response to disease is started by expression of cellular adhesion particles. Neutrophils are basic cell arbiters not just discharging proteolytic catalysts, but additionally producing responsive oxygen species, including myeloperoxidase (MPO), neutrophil elastase, and cathepsin G. Neutrophils discharge also neutrophil extracellular traps that instantiate extracellular chromatin threads with strong cytotoxic effects, containing both histones and granular proteins, which have bactericidal properties [57]. Also, neutrophil extracellular traps have prothrombotic properties, including activation of platelets, energizing of thrombin generation, and downregulation of anticoagulant pathways by the upgrade of APC resistance [58].

8. Diagnostic challenges of coagulopathy in sepsis

There are some totally different reasons for coagulation changes in septic patients. The reduced thrombocyte count is perpetually present in patients with serious sepsis; however, thrombocytopenia could likewise occur as a result of alternative conditions, for instance, immune thrombocytopenia (ITP), heparin-induced thrombocytopenia (HIT), thrombotic microangiopathies, or drug-evoked bone marrow distress [59]. It is critical to satisfactory pinpoint these different reasons for thrombocytopenia, as they may require specific administration projections [20]. Laboratory researches can be valuable in distinctive coagulopathy in sepsis from completely different alternative hemostatic conditions, such as vitamin K (vit K) bleeding or hepatic impairment. As these troubles might be observed simultaneously with sepsis-associated coagulopathy, dispersing is not in every case simple [60, 61].

As indicated by the contemporary pondering sepsis-associated coagulopathy, the evaluation of soluble fibrin in plasma has the mark of being significant [62]. Commonly, the affectability of measuring soluble fibrin for sepsis-associated coagulopathy is more optimal than the specificity. Some clinical assays have noted that at specific concentrations of soluble fibrin, sepsis-associated coagulopathy is highly tolerable [22]. Fibrin split products (FSPs) could be examined by specific Enzyme-Linked Immunosorbent Assay (ELISA) or by latex agglutination, enabling speed and bedside placement in very critical cases. None of the most accessible experiences for FDPs recognizes fragmentation products of cross-linked fibrin or fibrinogen degradation, which may contribute to faultily unusual results [53]. The specificity of elevated plasma levels of fibrin split products (FSPs) is subsequently unobtrusive, and a progression of other clinical circumstances, for example, trauma or injury, recent surgery, inflammation, or venous thromboembolism, may cause raised FDPs. More sophisticated tests specifically focus on the measurement of neo-antigens on fragmented cross-linked fibrin. Commonly, these measures respond with an epitope attached to plasmin-degraded cross-linked γ-chain, bringing about fragment D-dimer. These tests preferably identify the fragmentation of fibrin from fibrinogen (factor I) or fibrinogen degradation products (FDPs) [63]. Continuous coagulation activation brings exhaustion of coagulation factors in septic patients. Additionally, diminished synthesis, for example, brought by deranged hepatic function or vitamin K deficiency, and lack of coagulation factors, because of massive hemorrhage, might be significant. Estimation of plasma fibrinogen levels has been generally advanced as an accommodating tool for pinpointing coagulation anomalies in sepsis; yet in reality, this is not very supportive much of the time [10, 64]. Fibrinogen acts as an acute phase reactant, and regardless of impressive turnover, plasma concentrations can be well within normal values.

Thrombelastography is progressively utilized in critically sick patients with a hypercoagulable state, incorporating those with DIC [65, 66]. Procoagulant just as anticoagulant states in DIC as shown with thrombelastography was illustrated to have a better correlation with clinically significant organ dysfunction and survival despite the fact that its preference over usual coagulation tests has not yet been affirmed [67–72]. The precise utilization of thrombelastography for the conclusion of DIC has not been thoroughly assessed, despite the fact that supporters accept that the examiner might find it useful for evaluating the condition of coagulation in patients with critical sickness [73, 74]. In light of review investigations of databases from fundamentally sick patients, composite scores for the conclusion of sepsis-associated coagulopathy have been conceived by the International Society on Thrombosis and Hemostasis (ISTH) [75]. The system is in view of promptly accessible laboratory tests, that is, thrombocyte function, PT, D-dimer, and plasma fibrinogen levels. An analysis of DIC is perfect with a score of five or more excess points. PT manifested in seconds in the scoring order may be substituted by the INR, making symmetry among focuses and standardization simpler [76]. Approval investigations have demonstrated a high analytic precision of the scoring system [77, 78]. As a decision made a decision by this composite score is firmly connected with survival rates in climatically sick patients [79]. Joining predictive intensive care estimation systems, for example, Acute Physiology and chronic Health Evaluation (APACHE-II), with the DIC score is seemingly an intense technique to anticipate the prognosis in septic patients. Comparable composite scores are structured and examined in Japan [80]. The most applicable paradoxes between the ISTH and Japanese scores are a higher sensitivity and a higher extent of patients with hemato-oncological diseases that are determined to possess DIC by the Japanese systems [81, 82].

9. Conclusion

This work was basic elucidation of the idea that coagulation and its inhibitors are of major importance in coagulation-inflammation noise, similarly as in survival from sepsis. Further studies are warranted to explore the groundwork for the outcome of diagnostic rule victimization, many markers of inflammation and infection, and DIC score as parameters in assessing the severity of sepsis-associated coagulopathy in a clinical setting.

Author details

Bashir Abdrhman Bashir Mohammed

Address all correspondence to: bashirbashir17@hotmail.com

Faculty of Medical Laboratory Sciences, Port Sudan Ahlia College, Port Sudan, Sudan

References

[1] Angus DC, van der Poll T. Severe sepsis and septic shock. The New England Journal of Medicine. 2013;**369**(9):840-851

[2] Martin GS, Mannino DM, Eaton S, Moss M. The epidemiology of sepsis in the United States from 1979 through 2000. The New England Journal of Medicine. 2003;**348**(16): 1546-1554

[3] Angus DC, Linde-Zwirble WT, Lidicker J, Clermont G, Carcillo J, Pinsky MR. Epidemiology of severe sepsis in the United States: Analysis of incidence, outcome, and associated costs of care. Critical Care Medicine. 2001;**29**(7):1303-1310

[4] van der Poll T, van de Veerdonk FL, Scicluna BP, Netea MG. The immunopathology of sepsis and potential therapeutic targets. Nature Reviews. Immunology. 2017;**17**(7):407-420

[5] Levi M, van der Poll T. Coagulation and sepsis. Thrombosis Research. 2017;**149**:38-44

[6] Levi M. The coagulant response in sepsis. Clinics in Chest Medicine. 2008;**29**(4):627-642

[7] Gando S, Levi M, Toh CH. Disseminated intravascular coagulation. Nature Reviews Disease Primers. 2016;**2**:16037

[8] Levi M, ten Cate H. Disseminated intravascular coagulation. The New England Journal of Medicine. 1999;**341**(8):586-592

[9] Miller DL, Welty-Wolf K, Carraway MS, Ezban M, Ghio A, Suliman H, et al. Extrinsic coagulation blockade attenuates lung injury and proinflammatory cytokine release after intratracheal lipopolysaccharide. American Journal of Respiratory Cell and Molecular Biology. 2002;**26**(6):650-658

[10] Levi M, ten Cate H, van der Poll T. Disseminated intravascular coagulation: State of the art. Thrombosis and Haemostasis. 1999;**82**:695-705

[11] Ratnoff OD, Nebehay WG. Multiple coagulative defects in a patient with the Waterhouse-Friderichsen syndrome. Annals of Internal Medicine. 1962;**56**:627

[12] Wheeler AP, Bernard GR. Treating patients with severe sepsis. The New England Journal of Medicine. 1999;**340**(3):207-214

[13] Levi M, de Jonge E, van der Poll T. Sepsis and disseminated intravascular coagulation. Journal of Thrombosis and Thrombolysis. 2003;**16**(1-2):43-47

[14] Vanderschueren S, De Weerdt A, Malbrain M, Vankersschaever D, Frans E, Wilmer A, et al. Thrombocytopenia and prognosis in intensive care. Critical Care Medicine. 2000;**28**(6):1871-1876

[15] Strauss R, Wehler M, Mehler K, Kreutzer D, Koebnick C, Hahn EG. Thrombocytopenia in patients in the medical intensive care unit: Bleeding prevalence, transfusion requirements, and outcome. Critical Care Medicine. 2002;**30**(8):1765-1771

[16] Akca S, Haji Michael P, de Medonca A, Suter PM, Levi M, The VJL. Time course of platelet counts in critically ill patients. Critical Care Medicine. 2002;**30**:753-756

[17] Mavrommatis AC, Theodoridis T, Orfanidou A, Roussos C, Christopoulou-Kokkinou V, Zakynthinos S. Coagulation system and platelets are fully activated in uncomplicated sepsis. Critical Care Medicine. 2000;**28**(2):451-457

[18] Folman CC, Linthorst GE, van Mourik J, van Willigen G, de Jonge E, Levi M, et al. Platelets release thrombopoietin (Tpo) upon activation: Another regulatory loop in thrombocytopoiesis? Thrombosis and Haemostasis. 2000;**83**(6):923-930

[19] Francois B, Trimoreau F, Vignon P, Fixe P, Praloran V, Gastinne H. Thrombocytopenia in the sepsis syndrome: role of hemophagocytosis and macrophage colony-stimulating factor. The American Journal of Medicine. 1997;**103**(2):114-120

[20] Warkentin TE, Aird WC, Rand JH. Platelet-endothelial interactions: Sepsis, HIT, and antiphospholipid syndrome. Hematology. The Education Program of the American Society of Hematology. 2003;**1**:497-519

[21] MacLeod JB, Lynn M, McKenney MG, Cohn SM, Murtha M. Early coagulopathy predicts mortality in trauma. The Journal of Trauma. 2003;**55**(1):39-44

[22] Shorr AF, Thomas SJ, Alkins SA, Fitzpatrick TM, Ling GS. D-dimer correlates with proinflammatory cytokine levels and outcomes in critically ill patients. Chest. 2002;**121**(4):1262-1268

[23] Bernard GR, Vincent JL, Laterre PF, LaRosa SP, Dhainaut JF, Lopez-Rodriguez A, et al. Efficacy and safety of recombinant human activated protein C for severe sepsis. The New England Journal of Medicine. 2001;**344**(10):699-709

[24] Gando S, Nanzaki S, Sasaki S, Kemmotsu O. Significant correlations between tissue factor and thrombin markers in trauma and septic patients with disseminated intravascular coagulation. Thrombosis and Haemostasis. 1998;**79**(6):1111-1115

[25] Aird WC. Vascular bed-specific hemostasis: Role of endothelium in sepsis pathogenesis. Critical Care Medicine. 2001;**29**(7 Suppl):S28-S34

[26] Levi M, van der Poll T. Inflammation and coagulation. Critical Care Medicine. 2010;**38**(2 Suppl):S26-S34

[27] Taylor FB Jr, Chang A, Ruf W, Morrissey JH, Hinshaw L, Catlett R, et al. Lethal *E. coli* septic shock is prevented by blocking tissue factor with monoclonal antibody. Circulatory Shock. 1991;**33**(3):127-134

[28] Levi M, ten Cate H, Bauer KA, van der Poll T, Edgington TS, Buller HR, et al. Inhibition of endotoxin-induced activation of coagulation and fibrinolysis by pentoxifylline or by a monoclonal anti-tissue factor antibody in chimpanzees. Journal of Clinical Investigation. 1994;**93**(1):114-120

[29] Osterud B, Flaegstad T. Increased tissue thromboplastin activity in monocytes of patients with meningococcal infection: Related to an unfavourable prognosis. Thrombosis and Haemostasis. 1983;**49**(1):5-7

[30] Rauch U, Bonderman D, Bohrmann B, Badimon JJ, Himber J, Riederer MA, et al. Transfer of tissue factor from leukocytes to platelets is mediated by CD15 and tissue factor. Blood. 2000;**96**(1):170-175

[31] Zimmerman GA, McIntyre TM, Prescott SM, Stafforini DM. The platelet activating factor signaling system and its regulators in syndromes of inflammation and thrombosis. Critical Care Medicine. 2002;**30**(5 Suppl):S294-S301

[32] Shebuski RJ, Kilgore KS. Role of inflammatory mediators in thrombogenesis. The Journal of Pharmacology and Experimental Therapeutics. 2002;**300**(3):729-735

[33] Levi M, van der Poll T. Coagulation in patients with severe sepsis. Seminars in Thrombosis and Hemostasis. 2015;**41**(1):9-15

[34] Biemond BJ, Levi M, ten Cate H, van dP, Buller HR, Hack CE, et al. Plasminogen activator and plasminogen activator inhibitor I release during experimental endotoxaemia in chimpanzees: Effect of interventions in the cytokine and coagulation cascades. Clinical Science. 1995;**88**(5):587-594

[35] Hermans PW, Hibberd ML, Booy R, Daramola O, Hazelzet JA, de GR, et al. 4G/5G promoter polymorphism in the plasminogen-activator-inhibitor-1 gene and outcome of meningococcal disease. Meningococcal Research Group. Lancet. 1999;**354**(9178):556-560

[36] Westendorp RG, Hottenga JJ, Slagboom PE. Variation in plasminogen-activator-inhibitor-1 gene and risk of meningococcal septic shock. Lancet. 1999;**354**(9178):561-563

[37] Wiel E, Vallet B, ten Cate H. The endothelium in intensive care. Critical Care Clinics. 2005;**21**:403-416

[38] Keller TT, Mairuhu ATA, Kruif MD, et al. Infections and endothelial cells. Cardiovascular Research. 2003;**60**:40-48

[39] Szotowski B, Antoniak S, Poller W, et al. Procoagulant soluble tissue factor is released from endothelial cells in response to inflammatory cytokines. Circulation Research. 2005;**96**:1233-1239

[40] Osterud B, Bjorklid E. The tissue factor pathway in disseminated intravascular coagulation. Seminars in Thrombosis and Hemostasis. 2001;**27**:605-617

[41] Pawlinski R, Wang JG, Owens AP III, et al. Hematopoietic and nonhematopoietic cell tissue factor activates the coagulation cascade in endotoxemic mice. Blood. 2010;**116**:806-814

[42] Wagner DD. New links between inflammation and thrombosis. Arteriosclerosis, Thrombosis, and Vascular Biology. 2005;**25**:1321-1324

[43] Diamant M, Tushuizen ME, Sturk A, et al. Cellular microparticles: New players in the field of vascular disease? European Journal of Clinical Investigation. 2004;**34**:392-401

[44] Meziani F, Delabranche X, Asfar P, et al. Benchto-bedside review: Circulating microparticles—A new player in sepsis? Critical Care. 2010;**14**:236

[45] van der Poll T, Levi M, Hack CE, ten Cate H, van Deventer S, Eerenberg AJ, et al. Elimination of interleukin 6 attenuates coagulation activation in experimental endotoxemia in chimpanzees. The Journal of Experimental Medicine. 1994;**179**(4):1253-1259

[46] Stouthard JM, Levi M, Hack CE, Veenhof CH, Romijn HA, Sauerwein HP, et al. Interleukin-6 stimulates coagulation, not fibrinolysis, in humans. Thrombosis and Haemostasis. 1996;**76**(5):738-742

[47] Boermeester MA, van Leeuwen P, Coyle SM, Wolbink GJ, Hack CE, Lowry SF, et al. Interleukin-1 blockade attenuates mediator release and dysregulation of the hemostatic mechanism during human sepsis. Archives of Surgery. 1995;**130**(7):739-748

[48] Coughlin SR. Thrombin signalling and protease-activated receptors. Nature. 2000;**407** (6801):258-264

[49] Kaneider NC, Forster E, Mosheimer B, Sturn DH, Wiedermann CJ. Syndecan-4-dependent signaling in the inhibition of endotoxin-induced endothelial adherence of neutrophils by antithrombin. Thrombosis and Haemostasis. 2003;**90**(6):1150-1157

[50] Esmon CT. New mechanisms for vascular control of inflammation mediated by natural anticoagulant proteins. The Journal of Experimental Medicine. 2002;**196**(5):561-564

[51] Yuksel M, Okajima K, Uchiba M, Horiuchi S, Okabe H. Activated protein C inhibits lipopolysaccharide-induced tumor necrosis factor-alpha production by inhibiting activation of both nuclear factor-kappa B and activator protein-1 in human monocytes. Thrombosis and Haemostasis. 2002;**88**(2):267-273

[52] Murakami K, Okajima K, Uchiba M, Johno M, Nakagaki T, Okabe H, et al. Activated protein C attenuates endotoxin-induced pulmonary vascular injury by inhibiting activated leukocytes in rats. Blood. 1996;**87**(2):642-647

[53] Taylor FB Jr, Stearns-Kurosawa DJ, Kurosawa S, Ferrell G, Chang AC, Laszik Z, et al. The endothelial cell protein C receptor aids in host defense against Escherichia coli sepsis. Blood. 2000;**95**(5):1680-1686

[54] Levi M, Dorffler-Melly J, Reitsma PH, Buller HR, Florquin S, van der Poll T, et al. Aggravation of endotoxin-induced disseminated intravascular coagulation and cytokine activation in heterozygous protein C deficient mice. Blood. 2003;**101**:4823-4827

[55] Cohen J. The immunopathogenesis of sepsis. Nature. 2002;**420**:885-891

[56] Cross AS, Opal SM. A new paradigm for the treatment of sepsis: Is it time to consider combination therapy? Archives of Internal Medicine. 2003;**138**:502-505

[57] Xu J, Zhang X, Pelayo R, et al. Extracellular histones are major mediators of death in sepsis. Nature Medicine. 2009;**15**:1318-1321

[58] Ammollo CT, Semeraro F, Xu J, et al. Extracellular histones increase plasma thrombin generation by impairing thrombomodulin dependent protein C activation. Journal of Thrombosis and Haemostasis. 2011;**9**:1795-1803

[59] Baughman RP, Lower EE, Flessa HC, Tollerud DJ. Thrombocytopenia in the intensive care unit. Chest. 1993;**104**(4):1243-1247

[60] Levi M, de Jonge E, Meijers J. The diagnosis of disseminated intravascular coagulation. Blood Reviews. 2002;**16**(4):217-223

[61] Levi M, Toh CH, Thachil J, Watson HG. Guidelines for the diagnosis and management of disseminated intravascular coagulation. British Journal of Haematology. 2009;**145**(1):24-33

[62] Dempfle CE, Pfitzner SA, Dollman M, Huck K, Stehle G, Heene DL. Comparison of immunological and functional assays for measurement of soluble fibrin. Thrombosis and Haemostasis. 1995;**74**(2):673-679

[63] Horan JT, Francis CW. Fibrin degradation products, fibrin monomer and soluble fibrin in disseminated intravascular coagulation. Seminars in Thrombosis and Hemostasis. 2001;**27**(6):657-666

[64] Prisco D, Paniccia R, Bonechi F, Francalanci I, Abbate R, Gensini GF. Evaluation of new methods for the selective measurement of fibrin and fibrinogen degradation products. Thrombosis Research. 1989;**56**(4):547-551

[65] Shorr AF, Trotta RF, Alkins SA, Hanzel GS, Diehl LF. D-dimer assay predicts mortality in critically ill patients without disseminated intravascular coagulation or venous thromboembolic disease. Intensive Care Medicine. 1999;**25**(2):207-210

[66] Levi M, Meijers JC. DIC: Which laboratory tests are most useful. Blood Reviews. 2011;**25**(1):33-37

[67] Dempfle CE, Borggrefe M. Point of care coagulation tests in critically ill patients. Seminars in Thrombosis and Hemostasis. 2008;**34**(5):445-450

[68] Levi M, Hunt BJ. A critical appraisal of point-of-care coagulation testing in critically ill patients. Journal of Thrombosis and Haemostasis. 2015;**13**(11):1960-1967

[69] Johansson PI, Stensballe J, Vindelov N, Perner A, Espersen K. Hypocoagulability, as evaluated by thrombelastography, at admission to the ICU is associated with increased 30-day mortality. Blood Coagulation & Fibrinolysis. 2010;**21**(2):168-174

[70] Park MS, Martini WZ, Dubick MA, Salinas J, Butenas S, Kheirabadi BS, et al. Thromboelastography as a better indicator of hypercoagulable state after injury than prothrombin time or activated partial thromboplastin time. The Journal of Trauma. 2009;**67**(2):266-275

[71] Collins PW, Macchiavello LI, Lewis SJ, Macartney NJ, Saayman AG, Luddington R, et al. Global tests of haemostasis in critically ill patients with severe sepsis syndrome compared to controls. British Journal of Haematology. 2006;**135**(2):220-227

[72] Muller MC, Meijers JC, Vroom MB, Juffermans NP. Utility of thromboelastography and/or thromboelastometry in adults with sepsis: A systematic review. Critical Care. 2014;**18**(1):R30

[73] Brenner T, Schmidt K, Delang M, Mehrabi A, Bruckner T, Lichtenstern C, et al. Viscoelastic and aggregometric point-of-care testing in patients with septic shock–Cross-links between inflammation and haemostasis. Acta Anaesthesiologica Scandinavica. 2012;**56**(10):1277-1290

[74] Daudel F, Kessler U, Folly H, Lienert JS, Takala J, Jakob SM. Thromboelastometry for the assessment of coagulation abnormalities in early and established adult sepsis: A prospective cohort study. Critical Care. 2009;**13**(2):R42

[75] Taylor FB Jr, Toh CH, Hoots WK, Wada H, Levi M. Towards definition, clinical and laboratory criteria, and a scoring system for disseminated intravascular coagulation. Thrombosis and Haemostasis. 2001;**86**(5):1327-1330

[76] Kim HK, Hong KH, Toh CH. Application of the international normalized ratio in the scoring system for disseminated intravascular coagulation. Journal of Thrombosis and Haemostasis. 2010;**8**(5):1116-1118

[77] Bakhtiari K, Meijers JC, de Jonge E, Levi M. Prospective validation of the international society of thrombosis and haemostasis scoring system for disseminated intravascular coagulation. Critical Care Medicine. 2004;**32**:2416-2421

[78] Toh CH, Hoots WK. The scoring system of the scientific and standardisation committee on disseminated intravascular coagulation of the International Society on thrombosis and haemostasis: A five-year overview. Journal of Thrombosis and Haemostasis. 2007;**5**:604-606

[79] Dhainaut JF, Yan SB, Joyce DE, Pettila V, Basson BR, Brandt JT, et al. Treatment effects of drotrecogin alfa (activated) in patients with severe sepsis with or without overt disseminated intravascular coagulation. Journal of Thrombosis and Haemostasis. 2004;**2**:1924-1933

[80] Wada H, Gabazza EC, Asakura H, Koike K, Okamoto K, Maruyama I, et al. Comparison of diagnostic criteria for disseminated intravascular coagulation (DIC): Diagnostic criteria of the International Society of Thrombosis and Hemostasis and of the Japanese Ministry of Health and Welfare for overt DIC. American Journal of Hematology. 2003;**74**(1):17-22

[81] Wada H, Thachil J, Di NM, Mathew P, Kurosawa S, Gando S, et al. Guidance for diagnosis and treatment of DIC from harmonization of the recommendations from three guidelines. Journal of Thrombosis and Haemostasis. 2013;**11**:761-767

[82] Levi M. Settling the score for disseminated intravascular coagulation. Critical Care Medicine. 2005;**33**(10):2417-2418

Chapter 6

The Invariant Peptide Clusters of Serum Amyloid A Are Humoral Checkpoints for Vital Innate Functions as Probed by Monoclonal Antibodies, Including in Sepsis: Induction by Febrile Temperatures and Path of Discoveries

Reinhold P. Linke

Additional information is available at the end of the chapter

http://dx.doi.org/10.5772/intechopen.91983

Abstract

Serum amyloid A (SAA) is the most prominent acute-phase protein in vertebrates and its role in innate immunity has been reviewed. SAA functions are located on special regions of SAA, which are highly conserved in all vertebrates. 1. The discovery of the acute-phase nature of SAA before its existence was known by experimental murine AA amyloidosis induced by septic conditions. 2. Identification of the amyloid substance and its precursor. 3. SAA changes its conformation and antigenic presentation when it is separated from HDL during the acute phase. Febrile temperatures activate SAA through the separation from HDL. There is a temperature-specific gradual separation of SAA isotypes or groups of isotypes from HDL. 4. Generic monoclonal AA antibodies mc4 and mc29 assist in elucidating selected SAAs' vital functions (as in defense, platelet functions, female propagation and others). 5. In a murine sepsis model, the monoclonals mc4 and mc29 can cause early death while the intact SAA can prevent this. Through this, a checkpoint ("stop and go") for survival was discovered. Generic monoclonals can also identify the life-saving structures of SAA's vital functions and those of other acute-phase proteins. This principle is essential for the production of novel drugs against sepsis and other innate-related diseases. 6. Some remarks follow.

Keywords: amyloidosis, serum amyloid A (SAA), febrile temperatures, inflammations, sepsis, invariant checkpoints, generic monoclonal antibodies, innate immunity, therapeutic options

IntechOpen

1. The acute-phase nature of an enigmatic amyloid precursor in early experiments

1.1. Microscopic morphologic evidence

The task of my earliest work in pathology was to find out whether there was a soluble serum precursor for amyloidosis (This spacious scientific field has been reviewed pain part recently) [1, 2]. In experimental murine amyloidosis induced by septic conditions [3], morphologically significant signs are visible in **Figure 1** showing large amounts of hepatic amyloid (white areas), now recognized as amyloid A (AA). This amyloid was first deposited at the sites where the blood stream entered from the triangle of Glisson into the liver capillaries. The entire branches of blood vessels entering the liver parenchyma (left large vessel) are decorated with amyloid and, on the other hand, the branches that allow the blood to leave the liver are devoid of amyloid (right large vessel). This implies that the amyloidogenic protein is being deposited immediately when it reaches the liver upon assumed changing conditions (still unknown) by which amyloid is deposited from a soluble precursor. With time, the deposits grow by

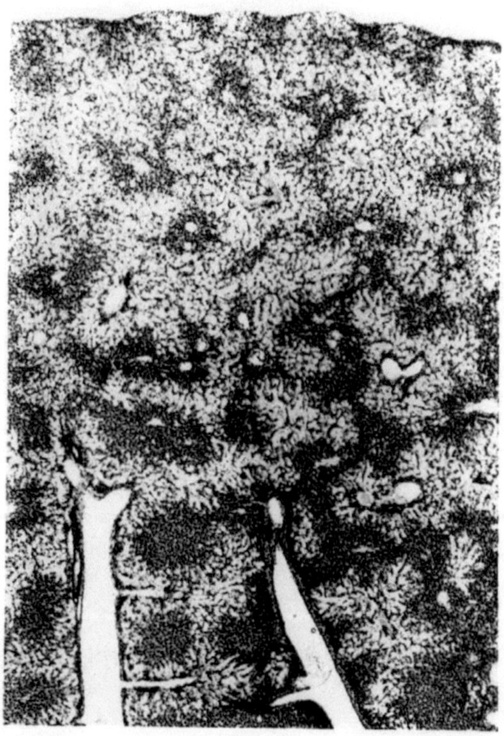

Figure 1. Photomicrograph of murine AA amyloidosis. Tissue section showing hepatic capillary amyloid deposits (white areas) induced by septic multi-microbial exposure after 25 days. The amyloid is deposited under pressure visible as the rough liver surface (at the top), which is usually sleek. Formalin-fixation, 4–6 μm paraffin section, HE-staining, magnification 24.1× [4].

apposition toward the central liver vein (darker areas) until most of the liver is transformed into amyloid in a fatal amyloidosis. This behavior requires a consistent, steady and very fast transformation of an assumed precursor to amyloid by entering the liver capillaries. The amyloid is deposited under pressure and visible as the rough liver surface (at the top), which is usually sleek.

1.2. Relative parabiotic barrier

When the assumed precursor is present in blood, as suggested by morphologic evidence, it should cross the anastomosis between artificial Siamese twins (parabiosis) with one partner induced to develop amyloidosis through septic conditions. However, this transmission does not always occur. The septic partner developed amyloid in 92.5% of pairs and the untreated partner in only 13.4%, and the latter was statistically not different to that seen in control pairs without any treatment [4]. The failure of crossing the anastomosis was excluded by ^{51}Cr-tagged erythrocytes [5]. Since the anastomosis was fully permeable, this type of parabiotic barrier was not an absolute one but a relative one caused by a short half-life of the agent that was removed from the bloodstream before it could cross the permeable anastomosis. The results of quantitation of the blood flow by ^{51}Cr erythrocytes, including a mathematical model of the exchange rate, shows that half of the blood was exchanged between the partners in 22.3 min. Therefore, a short half-life far below 22.3 min indicates a protein with a rapid clearance in minutes or even seconds, a property that is addressed today as an *acute-phase nature*, but still enigmatic precursor [5].

1.3. The clearance of SAA reported by other groups

The half-life of SAA1 and SAA2 in plasma of normal mice was reported for SAA-HDL as a T1/2 of 75–80 min and both isotypes were similar. However, when trace amounts of SAA were given, they were rapidly cleared [6]. Another report measured the clearance of the complex SAA-HDL for SAA1 T1/2 of 75 min and SAA2 T1/2 of 30 min, respectively. The clearance was delayed when both isotypes were bound to high-density lipoprotein (HDL) [7]. Both reports did not measure SAA under acute-phase conditions (APC). However, the report of Hoffman and Benditt [6] found a rapid clearance with trace amounts of SAA devoid of HDL and confirmed our data that are performed under a septic acute-phase condition that was to be observed when SAA was separated from HDL (see below).

2. Identification of the amyloid substance and isolation of its serum precursor

Amyloids of different clinical settings (also in animals, see **Figure 1**) represent characteristic fibrils under electron microscopy [8]. Therefore, for chemical identification of the amyloid, these fibrils had to be extracted in pure form followed by chromatographic isolation of the major amyloid protein for its chemical analysis by amino acid sequence analysis. The method of isolation of the pure amyloid fibrils was pioneered by Pras et al. [9]. The first amino acid sequence of an amyloid protein was published by Glenner et al. [10], which was derived from a monoclonal immunoglobulin κ-light chain and was named ALκ. The first sequence identifying the chemical nature of inflammation-induced amyloid in monkey and human amyloid was published by Benditt et al. [11], which was named amyloid A (AA). The first anti-AA antibodies were prepared in rabbits where a serum protein in patients suffering from inflammations was detected immunochemically. This protein had an α_1-electrophoretic mobility and was in serum approximately 180 KDa by calibrated gel filtration [12] and thus ready to monitor the isolation of the soluble with anti-AA reactive precursor. This isolation of serum protein began in summer 1972 and was monitored with another rabbit anti-AA antibody. Its chromatographic separation from serum yielded a native 200 ± 20 kDa AA reactive protein, which was further chromatographically isolated in 5 M guanidine-HCl. The AA reactive protein had an α_2-electrophoretic mobility and a molecular size of 12.5 kDa. Since this new protein had the same N-terminal amino acid sequence as AA, it was named serum amyloid A (SAA) [13]. Since SAA was larger than AA, a limited proteolytic cleavage had to be presumed in order for the former to generate AA. During the isolation of SAA and its purification to one size by gel filtration, by isoelectric focusing, however, eight SAA bands of different isoelectric point named A-H were identified with anti-AA antibodies (with AAE as the major SAA species for the planned radioimmunoassay), thus indicating the first signs of a polymorphism of SAA [13]. In addition, in plasma, SAA is bound to HDL [14].

3. SAA-HDL and febrile temperatures

3.1. Temperature-induced structural changes of SAA in serum

When examining a patient's acute-phase serum (APS) with elevated SAA in immunodiffusion (ID) at different temperatures and different times using a polyclonal AA antiserum in comparison with isolated control AA, this resulted in the three different precipitation patterns presented in **Figure 2**. In (a), one recognizes a line of identity of AA with all four patients' sera as if the SAA (probably SAA1 and SAA2) reaction were done with pure SAA. At 4°C in (b), however, there is no reaction with SAA-HDL in serum. This is due to the hiding of the AA-reactive parts of SAA through HDL. However, when the temperature was switched to room temperature after the reaction in (b) at 4°C the SAA containing serum resulted in a strong line after releasing the SAA from HDL in (c) as seen in (a). However, different from the pattern in (a), the precipitation line of AA-anti-AA is somewhat independent of the SAA-anti-AA line, thus indicating that the homologous AA-anti-AA line seems to be more stable than the SAA-anti-AA line. These results show that SAA-HDL is stable in full APS at 4°C where the AA-reactive sites are covered by HDL. When at room temperature (in ID buffer), where SAA is released from HDL and is now accessible to antibodies for precipitation, it is reactive. Therefore, the separation of SAA from HDL is temperature dependent [15]. These results became only fully explainable through Section 3.2, where the separation of SAA from HDL became clear [14].

In addition, we prepared recombinant SAA2 and, when added to normal human serum, it was possible to repeat exactly that behavior reported in **Figure 2**. This shows that SAA alone can reproduce this phenomenon [16].

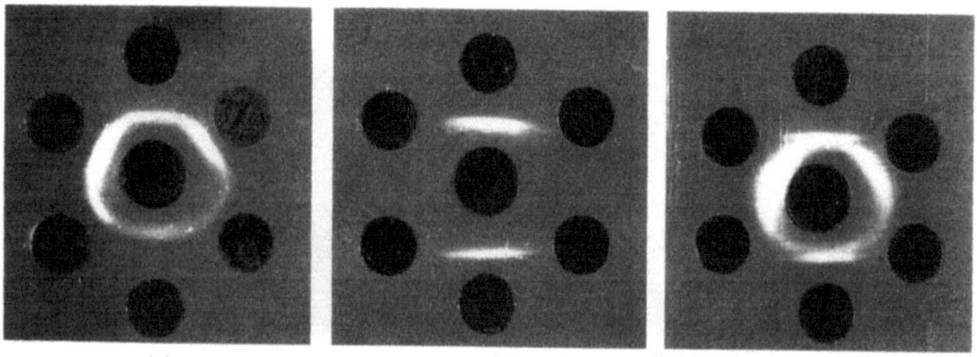

Figure 2. Immunochemical comparison of SAA-HDL, SAA and AA. Immunodiffusion (ID) at different temperatures [14, 15]. The ID was performed in 1.5% Seakem agarose in 0.03 M barbital buffer, pH 8.6 with the same reagents in each of the three plates à 6 wells ((a)-(c)). Top and bottom well contained AA (0.1 mg/ml), the middle well contained polyclonal rabbit anti-AA antibodies undiluted and the 4 side wells contained elevated SAA-HDL containing APS from 4 patients at 1/10 diluted. Plate (a) after diffusion over night at room temperature, plate (b) at 4°C over night and plate (c) first at 4°C over night as plate B at 4°C followed by room temperature for 6 h similar to plate (a).

3.2. The molecular size of the SAA and SAA-HDL at different febrile temperatures

Temperature-dependent molecular weight determination of AA-antigenic proteins of acute-phase serum (APS) has been performed using an ACA-34 gel filtration column in PBS with the enzyme inhibitor phenylmethylsulfonylfloride (PMSF) under various temperatures as shown in **Figure 3**. The size grading was done by the serum proteins IgM, IgG, albumin and, in addition, cytochrome C and the salt marker N-ε-DNP-lysine. The proteins were identified by way of the size position in the column by immunodiffusion as SAA-HDL at a size of ca. 180–200 kDa or SAA at 12.5 kDa. The different temperatures were kept with a temperature-controlled glass jacket, that is at 37°C in column run A, at 38°C in B, at 40°C in C and at 42°C in D. E was run as D, but without enzyme protection by PMSF, thus showing some degradation of SAA [18].

At a normal body temperature of 37°C, AA-containing proteins are at a single position as that of the SAA-HDL stable complex in A (fractions 34–37). However, already at 38°C, the stable complex SAA-HDL begins to dissociate as shown in **Figure 3**, run B. AA antigenic proteins appear at three positions, that is first of all at the void volume at fractions 19–20 (which has not been further analyzed, but could be related to aggregated SAA and/or its derivatives), secondly at the position of the stable SAA-HDL complex at fractions 34–36 and thirdly at the position of the HDL-free SAA at 53–56, as determined by the antigenic differentiation as seen in **Figure 2**. This size differentiation may also indicate functional heterogeneity, as the different affinities of SAA to HDL. This dissociation begins at 38°C and progresses with diminution of the SAA-HDL complex until run C. SAA-HDL disappeared at a "threshold of life" in run D at 42°C and above where the SAA species was maximized and the broadest was seen at fraction 53–56. This shows a temperature-induced gradual dissociation of SAA from HDL at the different febrile temperatures, which was shown here in vitro. This may also occur under systemic and local, acute-phase conditions, with the release of different SAA isotypes at different temperatures, for functions to be discovered. Finally, the SAA monomers released at different temperatures differ

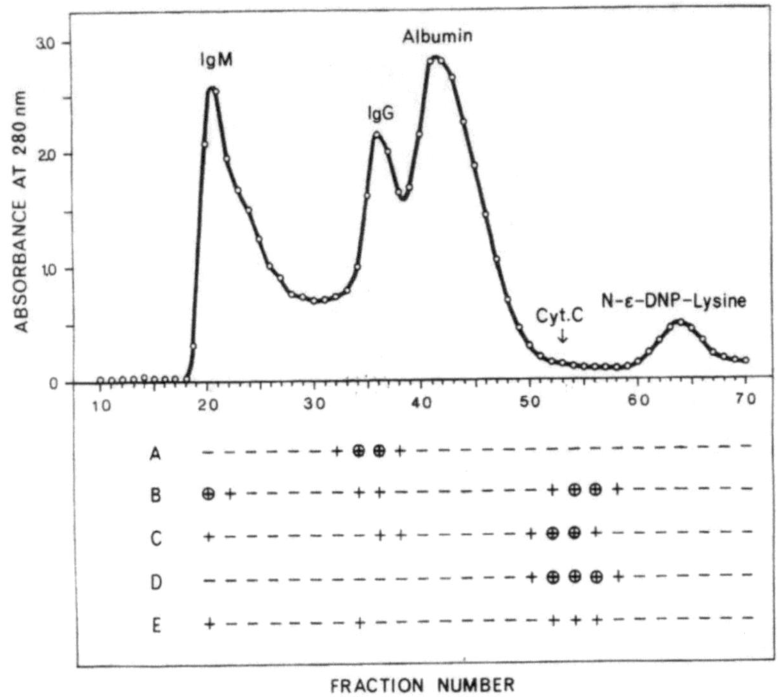

Figure 3. Size separation of SAA-HDL at febrile temperatures. SAA-HDL in a patient's acute-phase serum with a common cold was separated in A at 37°C, B at 38°C, C at 40°C and D at 42°C by gel filtration. All individual fractions (20–70) were examined and semi-quantified by ID using polyclonal rabbit anti-AA antibodies [15, 17].

in size. SAA in B is somewhat smaller than SAA in C. In addition, both appear at 42°C in D together as a broad combination of the two SAAs in B and D. In conclusion, SAA separated from HDL at 38°C in B has a lower affinity to HDL and is smaller, and SAA with a higher affinity for HDL is larger. Different isotypes and sizes of SAA are known [1, 2, 13]. The acute-phase SAAs, aSAA1 and aSAA2, are each 12.5 kDa with 104 amino acids and the constitutive SAA (cSAA), which is 14 kDa and has 112 amino acids. Since SAA1 has the lowest affinity for HDL and is the most amyloidogenic SAA, it could have separated from HDL in run at 38°C in B already, while SAA4, which is somewhat larger than the aSAAs, could be a component in the C. These indications can be solidified using isoelectric focusing or SAA-isotype-specific antibodies [1, 2].

3.3. Gradual dissociation of SAA-HDL during a continuous temperature gradient

While these experiments above were done stepwise, one by one, a more precise dissociation of the SAA-HDL separation was performed by electrophoresis in 1.5% agarose across a continuous temperature gradient in a single flat gel, as shown in **Figure 4**. The two sides between the agarose gel were kept at a constant temperature of 15°C in T1 and of 65°C in T2 [17].

The results in **Figure 4** show two horizontal bands of samples of one patient in the form of dots across the temperature gradient. The SAA-HDL band of α_1-electrophoretic mobility is marginally stained due to the concealing of the AA-antigenic determinants of SAA within

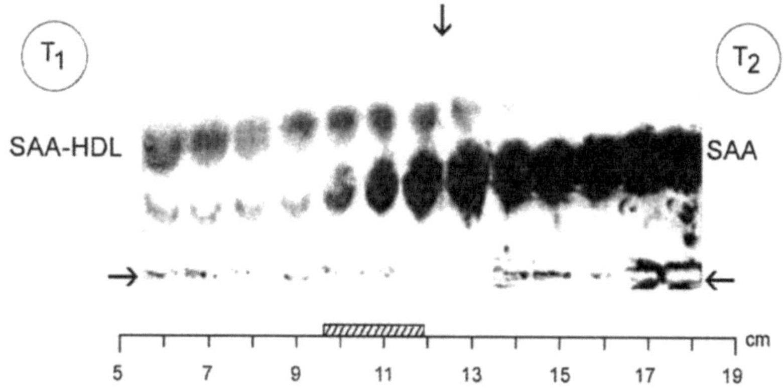

Figure 4. Electrophoresis of SAA-HDL across a continuous temperature gradient in agarose [18]. An APS was applied (see horizontal arrow) in 13 identical samples containing SAA-HDL across a temperature gradient. The small cross-hatched bar on the cm ruler denotes 37°C at the left margin and 42°C at the right one. Electrophoresis was done in 1.5% agarose (Seakem ME) in 25 mm barbital buffer, pH 8.6 followed by a standard Western blot developed with a mixture of the monoclonal anti-AA antibodies [19] mc1 + mc4 + mc29 at 1 + 1 + 1, 1/100 (see **Table 1**). One recognizes SAA-HDL at the left-side site marking the α_1-electrophoretic mobility (upper band). This band fades beginning from 38°C to 42°C, while the SAA freed from HDL (as in **Figure 3**) starts to appear at 38°C at the α_2-electrophoretic mobility with the very strong exposure of formerly concealed antigenic AA determinants detected after the strongest exposure appears at febrile temperatures between 38°C and 42°C (see cross-hatched bar). See vertical arrow at 42°C- 43°C.

the SAA-HDL complex at low temperatures. The hiding of the antigenic determinants disappeared gradually from 38°C (the 5th sample) until it is completely above 42°C with the appearance of large amounts of SAA (intensive staining of the band with α_2-mobility). By gradually increasing the temperature, the SAA release increases gradually while the SAA-HDL fades away up to the extreme exposure at 42°C and beyond, in agreement with the stepwise separation of SAA from HDL shown in **Figure 3**. Also important during this gradual temperature-induced separation from HDL seems to be that the morphology of the dots is different. They changed by their shape in the longitudinal direction, which is consistent with the fact that SAA is not uniform and consists of a group of homologous, but chemically different, SAAs demonstrating different isoelectric points (13 reviewed by [1, 2]). Another observation concerns the AA-antigenic species below 37°C in the first four samples. These slow, arc-like uniform samples could represent an SAA species, which is always active as a monomer regardless of temperature. This species seems to be less acidic. It could be a type of SAA species for the general protection under normal condition. In sample 5, this "arc SAA" is overlaid by a more acidic SAA released from the acute-phase proteins (APPs) SAA1 or SAA2, thus changing the spots to a more longitudinal pattern. With increasing temperature, the SAA spots become thicker and increase more in the longitudinal direction. This "arc SAA" needs to be analyzed since it does not seem to be part of the intact SAA-HDL complex (we did not check for SAA4). Finally, far above a temperature of 42°C, the SAA species seems to be stable. Parallel to the gradual release of SAA, at the same time, the SAA-HDL complex while losing SAA is gaining more negative charges with increased temperatures. Moreover, the trailing of SAA in samples 5–8 possibly indicates the gradual separation of differently charged SAA species.

3.4. Activation of the SAA by separation from HDL under febrile temperatures and consequences

Taken together [15, 17, 18, 21], it is clear that the mechanism of separation of SAA from HDL in vitro is also strictly regulated in vivo by body temperatures above 37°C. Therefore, this is a key mechanism that can be induced and activated basically by two different manifestations. The most common is the orthologic APR activation [33] of SAA. This occurs with a maximal SAA concentration of up to 1000 times within a day as a systemic "biochemical thunderstorm" with a myriad of activating and inhibiting events simultaneously, which are not understood in detail today [1, 2]. During these events, the cause of the APR will be eradicated and the APR becomes curative. With this beneficial outcome, the normal immune homeostasis returns in a foreseeable future. However, when the APR cannot overcome its initial cause, it will become a pathologic APR [33] with a "persistent biochemical thunderstorm" and lacking a self-driven cure. The consequences can be summarized in an exhaustion of the resources of the organism and decline of the metabolic activity through a multitude of clinically challenging conditions exemplified by severe viral and bacterial chronic inflammations, systemic inflammatory response syndrome (SIRS) or uncontrolled chronic infections, sepsis and septic shock [1, 2]. Moreover, when the infection remains limited, a local APR will take care of it.

The functions of the four human isotypes, SAA1, SAA2, (SAA3 in humans is only transcribed in some cells) and SAA4 have not been fully analyzed. They have arisen through gene duplications, thus indicating important individual functions either alone or in combination. As described before, the human acute-phase A-SAA has two very similar isotypes, A-SAA1 and A-SAA2, in the APR mostly synthesized in the liver and expressed in most body cells (see below) and the constitutive C-SAA4 and some allotypes in SAA1 and SAA2. For a review of the SAA heterogeneity and its known functions, see the reviews [1, 2].

Another discovery was the discontinuous separation of SAA from HDL described above at different temperatures, meaning that not all SAA molecules are being separated from HDL at a single temperature except for the temperature of 42°C (**Figures 3** and **4**). In fact, these figures show that the separation of SAA is spreading out over the whole febrile temperature range starting from 38°C to 42°C and above. In addition, based on these observations in **Figure 4**, it is possible that SAA isotypes and allotypes are separated from HDL at different febrile temperatures and thereafter fulfill their different functions locally or systematically as individual SAA species as is also to be derived from **Figure 3**. Another indication for the differential release of the SAA species can be detected in **Figure 4** in the different shapes of the protein blots of the SAAs devoid of HDL, thus indicating possible SAAs with distinct isoelectric points (IP). In **Figure 4**, there are free dots before 37°C named (for convenience) "arc SAA," the least acidic SAA. The SAA species released from HDL after 37°C ("38 SAA") are probably the more acidic ones. In this sense, the dot changes also occur later on 39°C-, 40°C-released SAA, etc. Analyzing the spots for the identity of the various SAA species could show whether these indications did discover a mechanism by which the different SAA species can be released from HDL and thereby are being activated at specific temperatures alone or with other SAAs for special purposes, which need to be analyzed. These points may also be of therapeutical interest. This proposed temperature selection of SAA isotypes could specify the needed APR function for a specific purpose. The increase of the organism's temperature is being induced by the organism as a response to various stimuli, exemplified by bacterial invasion. It could represent some sort of a "gear shift" for providing a graded response in order to release special SAAs to provide adequate amounts, which are necessary "tools" for survival. This could occur in concert with other agents including other APPs and cytokines of the APR network. The possible therapeutical manipulation of the body's temperature ("the gear shift") in vivo needs the precise analysis of this phenomenon in vivo first.

4. Application of antibodies

4.1. Polyclonal and monoclonal antibodies prepared against AA and SAA

In a collaborative study, each of the eight species-specific polyclonal AA antibodies against eight species (including humans) was immunohistochemically tested against the AA amyloids of eleven different species, including those of humans. The results showed a strong reactivity only with the homologous species and with only some cross-reaction with a related species. The reactivity was in general species specific, but a universal generic AA antibody could not be obtained in these eight polyclonal antibodies [37].

The next step was to produce murine monoclonal antibodies against AA and SAA [20]. Their value and merit have been documented by the inventors Köhler and Milstein [38]. Monoclonal antibodies are represented by one amino acid sequence and have the value of a chemical reagent. We selected 20 stable clones (see **Table 1**), which were epitope mapped [31] and immunohistochemically tested on AA amyloids in 10 different mammals, many humans and 9 different birds. Some cross-reactivity with some monoclonals was detected. Most of the 19 AA amyloids tested could be identified with the two monoclonals mc4 and mc29, showing that most of these AA amyloids have some peptides in common and these antibodies recognize the same or very similar epitopes of AA in different species. In addition, antibodies of all clones were tested for binding with 15 synthetic SAA peptides in only 4 clones the epitope could be identified. These included the known clones mc4 and mc29 (see above), and the two new ones, mc1 and mc20 (see **Table 1**). In APS, two different charge variants of SAA have been detected with these monoclonals [22].

The cause of the failing reactivity of most of the synthetic peptides with most of the monoclonals may be due to the presence of more discontinuous epitopes. This could also be deduced from the fact that SAA shows multiple short peptides that alternate between the invariable (red) and the variable (white) peptides, as shown in **Figure 5** (see also below).

Moreover, since mc21 was negative with the linear peptides, but reacted very strongly with AA amyloid in tissues, it was epitope mapped differently. It was mapped with endoproteinase Asp-N-generated peptides from a pure and partially amino acid-sequenced human AA (KIR) protein of 8.4 kDa. Of the 11 distinct peptides separated by RP-HPLC, mc21 reacted only with a single peptide, which was aa 33–42 of SAA [32]. This peptide is almost identical with the largest invariant peptide of SAA (see **Figure 5**). Two other monoclonals mc9 and mc13 did not show any reaction with these 11 distinct HPLC peaks [32] although they were reactive with AA in tissue sections. Here again, in linear SAA peptides, the discontinuous epitopes of SAA may not be preserved.

For notes	Clone no	Internal lab K-Nr.	Isotype	Quality			References (selected)
				Epitope and SAA peptides	Usage IHC	Usage EM	
	mc 1*	17	IgG 2a κ	5–16 7–15	+++	+++	[17, 20–28]
	mc 2				++		[22]
	mc 3	33			+		
	mc 4	34	IgG 1 κ	19–31	+++	+++	[17, 20–25, 29, 30]
	mc 8	38, 57	IgG 3 κ	25–76	++	0	[20, 22, 25]
	mc 9	39, 41, 53	IgG 1 κ		+++	0	[20, 22, 25, 31]
	mc 12	40, 42	IgG 2b κ	25–76	++	0	[20, 22, 25, 31]
	mc 13	43, 54	IgG 1 κ		+++	++	[20, 22, 24, 25]
	mc 15	45			+		
	mc 17	47			+		
	mc 20	50, 28 60	IgG 2a κ	60–75 25–76	++	+++	[17, 20–22, 25, 31]
	mc 21	65	IgG 1 κ	33-42	+++		[32]
	mc 22	70	IgG 2b κ		+	0	[25]
	mc 23	63	IgG 1 κ		+		
	mc 25	55, 124, 125, 126			++		
	mc 27	77, 127	IgM κ		++		
	mc 28	58, 128			+++	+	
	mc 29	129	IgG 1 κ	28–40 25–76	+++	+++	[17, 21, 24–31, 33–36]
	mc 30	130	IgG 1 κ		+++		
	mc 31	131	IgG 1 κ		+	0	[25]

Explanations: IHC, immunohistochemistry; EM, immunoelectron histochemistry.*Available from Dako, Denmark.

Table 1. Monoclonal AA and SAA antibodies [20].

Therefore, another strategy for the epitope mapping has been worked out that is the cooperative precipitation with either the antigens AA or SAA in 1.5% agarose gel. Applied were various combinations of two different monoclonals on one antigen, respectively. A precipitation showed that the two given monoclonals react with two epitopes. This approach resulted in precipitations and the epitope could be estimated roughly in some of the antibodies (unpublished). This has been expected since all the AA/SAA antibodies were selected by reactivity with amyloid in tissues. Finally, precipitation with SAA but not with AA pointed to a monoclonal against the SL peptide (see **Figure 5**, aa 77–104). Similarly, SAA isotype-specific monoclonals could have been selected by a similar approach.

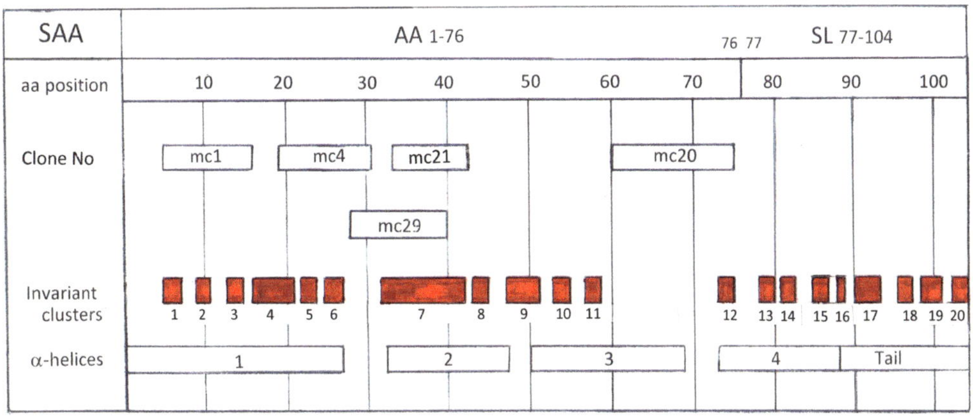

Figure 5. Structure of SAA and epitope-mapped AA monoclonal antibodies. The structure of SAA 1–104 and its fragments AA 1-76 and SL-77-104 with invariant (in red) and variant (white in between the red) peptides and epitope mapped of five monoclonal AA/SAA antibodies. There are three species-independent (mc4, mc21 and mc29), and two variant as well as species-specific (mc1 and mc20) monoclonal antibodies against AA and SAA. The positions of epitopes on the α-helical coils 1–4 and the contribution of the invariable (red) and variable peptides are also visible.

4.2. Identification of functional SAA epitopes by the monoclonals: finding their use and detecting their function

4.2.1. *Diagnostic application*

Monoclonals (see **Table 1**) are being applied for classification of AA amyloid in tissue sections when a recent amyloidosis was diagnosed in a patient or in an animal. Every amyloid has to be classified for therapeutic and prognostic purposes. This is exemplified in exploiting the generic monoclonals mc4 and mc29 (in Refs. [23, 24]) by either the immunohistochemical classification (IHC) on paraffin section of animal AA amyloidosis [23, 24] or by the immunoelectron microscopic classification (EM) of human AA amyloid on ultrathin sections [25].

4.2.2. *The structure of SAA*

The SAA1 and SAA2 proteins are presented in **Figure 5** as a continuous string with 1–104 amino acids. SAA consists of two parts, the N-terminal AA 1–76 polypeptide, which causes AA amyloidosis in humans [11] and animals under unfavorable inflammatory conditions [23, 24], and the C-terminal SL 77–104 polypeptide, whose function is stabilizing the two double coils [39, 40]. **Figure 5** was constructed using data from the USCS Genome Browser (GRCH38hg38) Assembly, as reported by 2.

The structure of SAA consists of four α-helical coils, 1–4, with 1–27, 32–47, 50–69 and 73–88 aa in length, respectively, followed by a tail after the 4th coil. These four coils are arranged in two antiparallel double coils, whereby 1 joins 3 and 2 joins 4 [39]. Each α-helix and its tail contain alternating blocks of twenty invariable peptides (**Figure 5**, in red, numbered 1–20). The variable peptides that can be species specific are the white, unstained sites in between the invariable peptides. Variables are also the peptides joining the coils, which represent the turns. In addition, the tail is winding around these double coils for stabilization [39, 40]. This conformation of SAA with the short-distance, alternating peptides in red and white would need more exact three-dimensional analyses for identifying the proposed discontinuities of peptides based on the partial un-reactivity of the monoclonals with linear peptides (see above).

4.2.3. The invariant peptide clusters of SAA and the binding sites of the SAA monoclonal antibodies

The monoclonal antibodies can be divided into three categories by the kind of epitope onto which they bind. In (a), they bind to species-specific epitopes and could perhaps also be detected with polyclonal antibodies [37]; in (b), they bind to AA amyloid in tissue section, but not to synthetic linear peptides, and are probably reacting with discontinuous epitopes of the SAA, and in (c), they bind to species independent, i.e., the invariant peptides and epitopes of AA and SAA, which are almost identical throughout the vertebrates (reviewed in [1, 2]). These special antibodies can also be called "generic" AA/SAA antibodies. Generic SAA antibodies are mc4, mc21 and mc29 (the latter contains also an additional specificity; see later). The two monoclonals that functionally bind to variable epitopes are mc1 and mc20 and belong to a category in (a). All monoclonals and their known binding synthetic peptides are listed in **Table 1**, together with their binding to patients' and animals' AA amyloid in formalin-fixed paraffin tissue sections [20, 23, 24] and ultrathin sections for EM [25].

The binding sites of the monoclonals to SAA are shown in **Figure 5**. The invariant parts of SAA contain ancient peptide clusters preserved during their evolution from the lampreys (over 500 Mio years without hardly any changes, Wikipedia) to the mammals, including humans. Again, we as humans have the invariable peptides of SAA in common with all vertebrates and the lamprey. Therefore, these special peptides have to be of utmost importance for mechanisms related to the proteostasis of many systems. They become extremely activated when in imbalance, exemplified by injuries and inflammation or bacterial infection, and in the event that their activation cannot be resolved. This can result in a sepsis. Thus, one can assume with some likelihood that a single amino acid exchange in these 19 invariant areas must not have been accepted throughout evolution. Indications are in the literature that natural SAA behaves differently as compared to recombinant SAA or SAA with a single amino acid change or exchange [1, 2]. The importance of the proteins of the SAA family for survival can therefore hardly be overestimated and the phrase that SAA is "the hub in the interaction network" [40] can express this eminent role of the SAA.

4.2.4. Properties of the individual monoclonals against AA presented here

4.2.4.1. mc1

This monoclonal antibody mc1 (see **Table 1** and **Figure 5**) is of interest since it binds to the most N-terminally positioned human-specific epitope on SAA (aa 5–16), but only when it is devoid of HDL. Thus, SAA can be distinguished from SAA-HDL through the failure of mc1 to bind to the complex of SAA-HDL, since HLD conceals the mc1 epitope of SAA [15].

Recombinant SAA shows the same binding to HDL and the same temperature release of SAA from HDL in vitro [21]. When separated from HDL under febrile temperatures, it can rebind again to HDL at body (or lower) temperatures. The binding is therefore reversible except when the temperature is above 41°C for some time, when it probably aggregates irreversibly [34]. The temperature-dependent mechanism has been proposed for activating the SAAs (see **Figures 2–4**). When fever is systemic, the free SAA load is part of the systemic APR. When local febrile temperatures are induced by local injuries or infection, a local APR is induced with local SAA. This can also apply for local tumors (see below). How this acts is not fully known. Where is the mc1 epitope located, considering that three invariant peptides are located within the 5–16 peptide stretch? Since the specificity is human specific, these peptides should be among the 2–3 variant areas; those are probably the white areas of the 5–16 peptide stretch; see **Figure 5**. In addition, this mc1 epitope (aa 5–16) has an overlap of 7 [5–11] of the 11 aa residues with the presumptive lipid-binding site (aa 1–11) (established by Turnell et al. [41]). Finally, mc1 binds very reliably to human (and some primate) AA in fixed paraffin sections and in ultrathin sections for EM [25], and not to SAA-HDL in serum at lower body temperatures (see above). Therefore, this murine monoclonal anti-AA mc1 has become a standard for examining human AA and SAA (available from Dako).

4.2.4.2. mc20

In tissue sections, this monoclonal (see **Table 1** and **Figure 5**) reliably binds to human AA amyloid and is being used for diagnostic purposes. It binds to the synthetic peptide aa 60–75 of SAA, which is located at the longest variable peptide stretch of SAA and located at the C-terminal half of the third α-helical coil, and, to a minor extent, at the small N-terminal part of the fourth coil, which contains the first invariable peptide no. 12. We do not know whether this mini peptide is part of the mc20 paratope.

4.2.4.3. mc4, mc21 and mc29

These antibodies demonstrated immunohistochemical, species-independent binding to most AA-type amyloids of the vertebrates (see above). They were therefore directed against the invariant peptides of SAA, which are located on the first and second α-helical coils. Their extent and their differences are depicted in **Figure 5**. The clone mc4 reacts largely with the invariant peptide no. 4–6 on coil 1. This clone binds differently as compared to mc21 and mc29, both of which bind to the 7th peptide of coil 2, the largest invariant peptide of SAA. While mc21 seems to be only reacting with peptide no. 7, the monoclonal mc29 extends to the variant joining peptide area (aa 28–32) that is between coil 1 and coil 2. This may explain the additional, partial binding of mc29 to the variable peptides. In addition, it binds to most of the animal AA amyloids tested (see below).

4.2.4.4. mc1, mc4, mc13, mc29 and mc31

This series of monoclonal antibodies has been probed and exerted to establish a monoclonal micro-ELISA for quantification of SAA [42].

5. On SAAs' functions and their identification by blocking the invariant epitopes of SAA

5.1. The multifunctional SAA family

Various functions of SAA have been reported, including the systemic and local elevation of SAA in inflammations in an APR due to the systemic and local cytokine increase. SAA is involved in very many functions as being an opsonin of Gram-negative bacteria, a chemoattractant, an inducer of chemokines and cytokines, a stimulator of angiogenesis, important in cholesterol transport and a modulator in the migration of white blood cells. SAA acts concentration dependently on polymorphonuclear cells and the degradation of SAA (by matrix degradation enzymes?), which can release the AA 1–76 fragment and can thereby induce the fatal AA amyloidosis in humans and animals. Other fragments of SAA and other APPs may, in vivo, influence this still not understood complex network of the SAA family, which has been reviewed in [1, 2, 43, 44]. Here, some of these vital functions of SAA have been identified by blocking these functions by way of monoclonal AA/SAA antibodies. At the same time, the SAA binding motives have been localized at the surface of SAA (see **Figure 5**). Alternatively, these ligands for the SAA binding motives can, in part, be blocked with the respective synthetic peptides of SAA [44, 45].

5.2. HDL binding site

The HDL binding site of SAA was identified as the peptide aa 5–17 with the monoclonal mc1 (see Section 4). The presumptive estimate by Turnell et al. [41] was aa 1–11.

5.3. Human neutrophils

Strong binding of isolated, acute-phase human SAA (and recombinant SAA2, not presented) were shown with human neutrophils [33] assuming the existence of an SAA receptor, which may have regulatory functions [1, 2]. The FMLP-induced oxidative burst of normal human neutrophils could be reduced, concentration dependently, by SAA at concentrations of 0.1 μg/ml and 1.0 μg/ml. This inhibitory reduction of SAA could be blocked by the monoclonal antibody mc29 (see **Table 1** and **Figure 5**), which binds to the synthetic peptide aa 28–40 of SAA, thus proving that this blocked area is responsible for this inhibitory effect of SAA [33]. This was the first time that a function of SAA was blocked by a monoclonal AA antibody. Moreover, at the same time, the responsible peptide of SAA was identified, which was the invariant peptide no. 7 of coil 2. The monoclonal antibody mc29 used probably also blocks the laminin-like domain (aa 29–33) and may also be participating partially with the RGD-like domain (aa 39–41). In addition, human neutrophils were exposed to full human APS at different temperatures [34]. At 41°C, the inhibition of the oxidative burst was much stronger than at 37°C, indicating the role of SAA freed from HDL and in its active state (see Section 3.4; see **Figures 3** and **4**). However, when the acute-phase serum was preheated to 41°C for 15 min and assayed at 37°C, the SAA-containing serum did not return to the 37°C value, but stayed with the increased 41°C inhibiting effect at 37°C. This indicated an irreversible structural change of SAA (or its fragments) during high fever, which is blocking SAA's return to the reversible binding to HDL. (This febrile temperature that induced the aggregation of AA-antigenic proteins has also been noticed in vitro and documented in **Figure 3** at 38°C and 40°C). The possibly unfavorable consequences of these aggregates in humans or animals are unknown today.

5.4. Anti-inflammatory potential of SAA on neutrophils

The anti-inflammatory potential of SAA on neutrophils [33] has been confirmed for SAA at reported serum concentrations [46]. Oxidative burst, migration and the neutrophil myeloperoxidase release were also inhibited. SAA peptides (aa 1–14, 15–101 and 83–104) also contributed to this inhibitory effect. However, at higher concentrations of more than 50 μg/ml, SAA was stimulating. In addition, O_2 release was inhibited up to 0.1 μg/ml, but the O_2 release was increased above that. Thus, SAA plays a dual role, it downregulates inflammatory processes in lower concentration, but, during the full APR, the action of SAA can be promoting.

5.5. SAA functions inhibited by synthetic peptides

SAA functions can be identified by SAA-generic antibodies [33, 34, 46] but they can also be blocked by synthetic peptides of SAA [45]. This was shown through the use of a 14mer synthetic peptide (aa 29–42) of SAA. This peptide inhibited the binding of T lymphocytes and mouse M4 melanoma cells to adhesive glycoproteins of the extra cellular matrix. This SAA 14mer peptide contained the laminin-like (aa 29–33) and fibronectin-like (aa 13–15) domains of the extracellular matrix. Finally, by extending these data of the 14mer SAA peptide, by comparing to the binding of our generic antibodies mc21 and mc29, it is to be said that these antibodies bind to a similar peptide of SAA, which is the largest invariable peptide (no. 7 of coil 2) as shown in **Figure 5**.

5.6. Phagocytosis

Phagocytosis was examined on fixed bacteria by normal and stimulated blood monocytes at the SAA concentration that were inhibitory to human neutrophil activation [33]. There was no difference in phagocytosis in the presence or in the absence of SAA [47].

5.7. Platelets and binding motives similar to SAA

Human platelet adhesion was shown to immobilize SAA and the mechanism of binding was examined [35]. Among the many receptors on platelets, the receptors for laminin and fibronectin were chosen to be examined because SAA has laminin-like and fibronectin-like motives in its sequence. Immobilized SAA binds platelets as do fibronectin and, to a lesser degree, fibrinogen. This binding of SAA to platelets was completely abolished by anti-SAA (mc29), which binds to the laminin-like motive on SAA (aa 29–33) that is part of the mc29-binding peptide. Also, a 29–42-containing peptide could inhibit the binding of platelets to SAA. In addition, an antibody against an integrin receptor also inhibited the binding as well the RGD-containing peptide GRGDSP. Also, the anti-SAA (mc29) did not inhibit the RGD-dependent binding motive to a significant extent, thus indicating that the overlap of two amino acids (aa 39–40) of the peptide (see **Figure 5**) did not lead to an efficient paratope subsite of mc29 for the method applied. Finally, all controls were in line with the conclusion that SAA was binding to platelets via the laminin-like and fibronectin-like motives. Since the related binding motives are not chemically identical with laminin or fibronectin, they could have a lower affinity, which may be exerted differently at lower concentrations as compared with higher concentrations, i.e., during the APR.

Thus, SAA may play a role in inhibiting and modulating platelet adhesion at vascular injury sites by sharing platelet receptors with other platelet-adhesive proteins. In addition, depending on the kind of disease, the window between bleeding and thrombosis may sometimes be very narrow; how can it be widened? Finally, systemic and local thrombosis are not rare, which are life-threatening sequels of many conditions. These are related to arteriosclerosis, heart conditions, nutrition-related ailments, deranged lipid metabolism, smoking and other drugs, cancer, injuries, bacterial infections and sepsis, mostly in a more advanced age as well as in cases of vascular injury. The role of platelets is central in these and many other diseases, and the concentration-dependent role of SAA and its antidotes (humanized monoclonals and others) in vivo needs to be explored and then further developed.

5.8. Presence of SAA in human cancer and other cells

Intracellular SAA of colon tissue with cancer of progressing stages of anaplasia was examined on formalin-fixed paraffin sections from 26 patients with colon cancer (after SAA plasma levels were shown by others to be elevated in carcinomas, assuming that the elevated SAA is of hepatic origin) [26]. SAA was detected immunohistochemically by using the monoclonal antibodies mc1 and mc29 (specificity, see **Figure 5** and **Table 1**). On normal cells, no reaction or only traces were detected. However, stronger reactions were found in carcinoma cells. The staining intensity increased gradually from dysplasia to the stage of malignant neoplasia. The metastases also showed the presence of SAA, but weaker. In addition, cells, other than colon cells in these sections, also showed the presence of SAA as lymphoid cells of the intestinal wall, inflammatory cells, ganglion cells and endothelial cells. The presence of SAA has been confirmed by in situ hybridization and reverse transcriptase polymerase chain reaction (RT-PCR). The genes of SAA1 and SAA4 in the colon carcinomas were activated. Although the role of SAA in colon carcinoma is unknown, the close association of the increasing grade of malignancy with the increased SAA synthesis may indicate a role of SAA in tumorigenesis. SAA can serve as an adhesive ligand for tumor-cell homing; it induces inflammation, which may be neoplastic. It also induces migration and can be involved in metastasis, or it can be inhibitory to attachment [26].

5.9. Protein SAA enhances plasminogen activation and may contribute to tumor spread

The colon carcinoma cell line HT-29 showed plasminogen activity (PA) enhanced by SAA measured with a chromogenic substrate. This activity could be inhibited using monoclonal antibodies against SAA (mc1 + mc29). The cell line also produced endogenous SAA1 by itself, which could be augmented by exogenous SAA and also by cytokines IL-1b and IL-6. This activity was also inhibited in part by the monoclonal antibodies against SAA [36]. The concomitant overexpression and co-localization of SAA and PA in colon cancer cells raises the possibility of a functional relationship between these two systems. The authors suggest that SAA produced in the malignant tissue may contribute to increased matrix degeneration and tumor spread [36].

5.10. Gradual increase of SAA while progressing to malignancy in ovarian epithelial tumors

Increased levels of SAA were reported in a wide range of malignancies, as well as another unspecific tumor marker, with an increase in metastatic tumors and regression when therapy is successful [26]. Here, the presence of SAA in serum (with CRP and CA-123) and expressed locally in tissues was examined and compared with different stages of tumor growth. Compared were normal ovarian tissues, benign, borderline, carcinoma and metastatic tissues of patients using immunohistochemistry with monoclonal antibodies against AA (mc1 and mc29, see **Table 1** and **Figure 5**) and in situ hybridization. In some patients (and in cell line OVCR-3), RT-PCR was applied, and SAA1 and SAA4 were detected. The result shows a continuous increase of SAA (CRP and CA-125) in serum during the gradual increase of the malignant nature of the ovarian tissue proliferation. In addition, and most important, the SAA expression in tissue increases, in the same manner, with a steep increase in the SAA-synthesizing cells from the normal cells, without (or with only a trace of) SAA, over the borderline tumors with weak expression to the maximal expression of the distinct carcinomas and metastases. Therefore, it is likely that the serum level of SAA in these malignancies may, in part, originate from the ovarian tumor itself.

The data show that the quantity of local intracellular expression of SAA correlates directly with the grade of malignancy of the ovarian epithelial neoplasias and runs in parallel with the serum value of SAA, CRP and CA-125. Therefore, SAA may have a role in ovarian tumorigenesis [27].

5.11. SAA in the female reproductive system

Ovarian reproduction includes a kind of inflammatory process [28]. Therefore, the cellular expression and localization of SAA in all stages of follicular development was examined in in vitro fertilization (IVF) patients applying nonradioactive in situ hybridization and immunochemistry with the monoclonal anti-AA (mc1 and mc29) antibodies. In parallel, SAA of follicular fluids and SAA in serum were examined using micro-ELISA. Expression of SAA mRNA was found in all follicular cells (granulosa, thecal and luteal) of all stages of development, from primordial, primary and secondary follicles to corpora lutea and even in oocytes.

The concentration of SAA in serum and in the matched follicular fluid was very closely associated ($R^2 = 0.80$), although both values could vary considerably by a factor of ca. 30× for blood SAA and by 100× for the follicular fluid. In addition, elevated follicular SAA values have a strong correlation with the patients' body mass index. Values over 30 are associated with a reduced pregnancy rate. Taken together, SAA is locally produced by all follicular cells and is a constituent of the follicular fluid. Therefore, it has a role in ovarian development and in the rate of pregnancy, which is reduced when SAA values are too high in overweight female patients with a BMI of over 30.

Finally, since human ovarian epithelial tissues reproduce SAA during reproduction (see above), the neoplastic degenerated cells in ovarian carcinoma continue their SAA synthesis [26].

5.12. A role of SAA in the APR of murine septic inflammations

5.12.1. On the role of the APR and APPs in septic mice

In order to analyze the different steps necessary to overcome an infection by the hepatic APR, an experimental mouse model was applied and shown as an "anti-sepsis circle" (see **Figure 6**) [32]. Using polymicrobial sepsis induced by cecal ligation and puncture (CLP), the various actions begin with mice exposed to a bacterial overload that leads to the IL-6 induction, which is the dominant interleukin and major inductor of the APR. IL-6-deficient mice can still mount an APR, since IL-6 represents one member of a larger group of interleukins with redundant actions. The action of IL-6 is to initiate the intracellular signaling via the hepatic IL-6 receptor gp130 and further induction of STAT3, which is inevitable for developing the full hepatic APR in hepatic cells, including the synthesis of the dominant APP SAA. However, when mice with a deletion of gp130 or STAT3 are treated with CLP, the hepatic synthesis of SAA is not induced and these mice cannot mount an APR anymore and are thus defenseless, and mortality is greatly increased. The missing APR and the missing defense can be reversed by adding myeloid-derived suppressor cells (MDSCs), which are induced by a hepatic APR including SAA. SAA induces and activates the proliferation of bone marrow cells, which include MDSCs. These cells are accepted to be able to also act against the microbial infection. MDSCs are anti-inflammatory in cancer, cancer spread and metastases [27]. They home-in on different organs. In septic mice, they have been examined from spleen and increase their numbers when pg130 and STAT deficiency are overcome by an

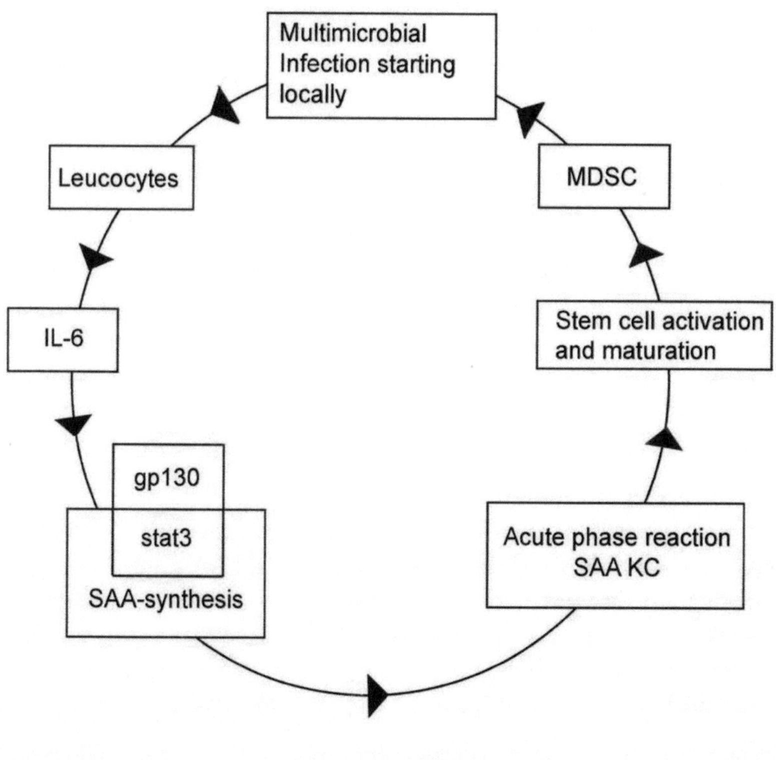

Figure 6. Closing the sepsis loop to the "anti-sepsis circle" schematically.

injection of SAA, cxcl (KC) or SAA/KC. MDSC can be regarded as a second anti-inflammatory wave induced by SAA and the other components of the APPs when the first wave of anti-inflammatory phagocytes is beginning to wane while becoming exhausted [1, 2, 27].

When very important functions of SAA (which need to be more clarified) are being blocked by the monoclonal antibodies mc4 and mc29 in CLP mice, the essential MDSCs cannot be produced to the necessary amount and function to cope with the bacterial load so that the mice become defenseless and display a significantly accelerated death rate. This unfavorable situation can be reverted by the injection of SAA, thereby resulting in the former defense with the proliferation of MDSCs, so that the mice survived like CLP-treated mice in this sepsis model [29, 30, 48]. The APP KC has a similar, but not identical, effect. When KC was added to SAA, the recovery from the CLP fate of mice with a murine SAA inactivated by antibodies may even be slightly improved, thus indicating that SAA, although the major and dominant APP, can be assisted by KC against the bacterial load.

This demonstrates a cooperative defense of SAA and KC [29]. Cooperation can also be expected from other APPs and constituents in the APP network, including from the greater SAA family. The AA antibodies mc4 and mc29 bind to invariant and therefore very important peptides of SAA as described in detail in Section 4.2, in **Table 1** and **Figure 5**. With these antibodies, life-saving biological functions have been detected and their functions localized to invariant peptides of SAA. This approach could be extended to analyze all the invariant peptides of the SAA family. This can be regarded as a starting point for a possible therapy of a long list of such maladies as severe chronic inflammations and severe chronic infections including sepsis with (induced in vivo or recombinant) SAA isotypes (and their inhibitors as humanized generic SAA antibodies), and with other APPs and constituents of the network of the SAA family, which are able to fortify the "anti-sepsis circle" (**Figure 6**).

6. Some remarks

6.1. The septic loop became an "anti-sepsis circle" as a basis for further work

Some essential elements of the cooperative defense against the experimental multi-microbial infections became apparent as shown in **Figure 6**. The pathway from infection procedures passes, through IL-6, gp130 and STAT3, to the APR with the dominant SAA family and its network. This loop has been closed to a circle through the action of at least the SAA1 that assisted in inducing the growth of the MDSCs in the bone marrow. These cells are also shown to be essential in fighting bacterial infection. However, when gp130 or SAA was not available in this model and the "circle" was interrupted, with fatal consequences, the addition of the missing agents restored the circle with its function [29]. It should be an important goal to examine the SAA isotypes in different inflammatory states and diseases in relation to febrile temperatures (**Figures 3** and **4**) and to analyze the functions of all 20 invariant peptides (**Figure 5**) and the epitopes of the AA/SAA antibodies (**Table 1**) in order fortify it.

It is also important to define the febrile temperatures by which the individual SAAs separate from HDL (proven in vitro, **Figures 3** and **4**) and get activated to execute their function. A novel idea could be: therapeutical hypothermia below 37°C could inactivate SAA through binding to HDL, which can be called "hypothermic deactivation of SAA." This option could be considered (after complying with the strict rules for a novel therapy) in severe inflammatory states exemplified by sepsis, septic shock, genetic hyperthermia syndromes and similar diseases summarized in SIRS (systemic inflammatory response syndrome). Inversely, a temperature-dependent conformational change of SAA at above 38°C causing SAA release from HDL can induce a "hyper-thermic activation of SAA," which could be beneficial for patients having clinical syndromes with body temperatures of 36°C and below.

6.2. Innate, humoral checkpoints for survival and application by industrial organizations

The presented view summarizes peptides of SAA that are decisive for innate humoral functions in different systems. This view can be applied to many possible possible inflammatory and infectious diseases, including sepsis. These SAA peptides provide a functional innate humoral "stop and go" mechanisms located on SAA ("SAA checkpoints") related to survival. Stop, with generic (humanized) AA/SAA monoclonal antibodies or equivalent agents, and go, with the bio-identical SAA preparations, including SAA isotypes or related peptides with special SAA functions (**Figure 5**), which need to be further explored to find out their additional role in the SAA network. This examination can also be extended to other APPs.

6.3. European Patent EP No 2368564

Due to its novelty within the field of innate immunity and the possibly far-reaching impact in medicine, in particular, in inflammatory diseases including sepsis, these discoveries by three inventors were in agreement with the two other inventors patented by the author [49, 50].

Acknowledgement

For help with the figures, I thank Ms. Anne Linke, Zürich, Switzerland.

Dedication

This chapter is dedicated to Professor Dr. Konrad Beyreuther, Heidelberg and Professor Dr. Robert Huber, Martinsried, Germany.

Author details

Reinhold P. Linke

Address all correspondence to: linke@amymed.de

Max-Planck-Institut für Biochemie, Martinsried, Germany

References

[1] De Buck M, Gouwy M, Wang JM, Van Snick J, Opdenakker G, Struyf S, et al. Structure and expression of different serum amyloid A (SAA) variants and their concentration-dependent functions during host insults. Current Medicinal Chemistry. 2016;**23**(17): 1725-1755

[2] Sack GH. Serum amyloid A—A review. Molecular Medicine. 2018;**24**(1):46. DOI: 10.1186/s10020-018-0047-0

[3] Linke RP. The experimental production of amyloidosis. Zeitschrift für die Gesamte Experimentelle Medizin. 1969;**150**:150-160

[4] Linke RP, Kuni H. Transmission studies of amyloidosis by parabiosis of isogeneic mice. Virchows Archiv A Pathological Anatomy and Histology. 1969;**346**:89-102

[5] Linke RP, Kuni H, Wechselberger H. Quantitative determination of cross circulation in parabiosis of isogeneic mice. Zeitschrift für die Gesamte Experimentelle Medizin. 1969;**149**:152-165. Available from: https://www.ncbi.nlm.nih.gov/pubmed/5384951

[6] Hoffman JS, Benditt EP. Plasma clearance kinetics of the amyloid-related high density lipoprotein apoprotein, serum amyloid protein (apoSAA), in the mouse. Evidence for rapid apoSAA clearance. Journal of Clinical Investigation. 1983;**71**(4):926-934

[7] Kluve-Beckerman B, Yamada T, Hardwick J, Liepnieks JJ, Benson MD. Differential plasma clearance of murine acute-phase serum amyloid A proteins SAA1 and SAA2. Biochemical Journal. 1997;**322**(Pt 2):663-669

[8] Cohen AS, Calkins E. Electron microscopic observations on a fibrous component in amyloid of diverse origins. Nature. 1959;**183**(4669):1202-1203. No abstract available

[9] Pras M, Zucker-Franklin D, Rimon A, Franklin EC. Physical, chemical, and ultrastructural studies of water-soluble human amyloid fibrils. Comparative analyses of nine amyloid preparations. Journal of Experimental Medicine. 1969;**130**(4):777-796

[10] Glenner GG, Harbaugh J, Ohma JI, Harada M, Cuatrecasas P. An amyloid protein: The amino-terminal variable fragment of an immunoglobulin light chain. Biochemical and Biophysical Research Communications. 1970;**41**(5):1287-1289. No abstract available

[11] Benditt EP, Eriksen N, Hermodson MA, Ericsson LH. The major proteins of human and monkey amyloid substance: Common properties including unusual N-terminal amino acid sequences. FEBS Letter. 1971;**19**(2):169-173

[12] Levin M, Pras M, Linke RP, Franklin E. Immunologic studies of ASF, the major nonimmunologic component of certain amyloid fibrils. Arthritis and Rheumatism. 1973;**16**:123

[13] Linke RP, Sipe JD, Pollock PS, Ignaczak TF, Glenner GG. Isolation of a low-molecular-weight serum component antigenically related to an amyloid fibril protein of unknown origin. Proceedings of the National Academy of Sciences of the United States of America. 1975;**72**(4):1473-1476

[14] Benditt EP, Eriksen N. Amyloid protein SAA is associated with high density lipoprotein from human serum. Proceedings of the National Academy of Sciences of the United States of America. 1977;**74**(9):4025-4028

[15] Linke RP. Antigenic difference between serum amyloid protein SAA and its low molecular weight derivative SAAL revealed by an anti-amyloid A antiserum at different temperatures. Zeitschrift für Immunitätsforschung. Immunobiology. 1978;**154**(2):169-172

[16] Noetzel F, Frankenberger B, Haindl E, Linke RP. Comparison of recombinant and native serum amyloid A protein with regard to lipoprotein binding using a panel of monoclonal antibodies. In: Kyle RA, Gertz MA, editors. Amyloid and Amyloidosis. New York, London: Parthenon Publ. Group; 1999. pp. 378-38

[17] Linke RP. Immunochemical investigation on serum amyloid A (SAA): Temperature-induced changes of its quaternary structure. In: Glenner GG, Costa PP, Freitas AF, editors. Amyloid and Amyloidosis, Excerpta Medica. Amsterdam; 1980. pp. 313-319

[18] Linke RP. Temperature-induced dissociation of serum amyloid protein SAA. Zeitschrift für Immunitätsforschung. Immunobiology. 1979;**155**(3):255-261

[19] Linke RP. Two different sets of charge variants of amyloid fibril protein AA recognized by monoclonal antibodies. Protides of the Biological Fluids. 1986;**32**:387-390

[20] Geisel O, Linke RP. Generalized AA-amyloidosis in two hares (Lepus europaeus) immunohistochemically identified using poly- and monoclonal antibodies. Veterinary Pathology. 1988;**25**(5):391-393

[21] Frankenberger B. Das Akutphasenprotein Serumamyloid A: Isolierung von Isotypen, Epitopkartierung mit Hilfe monoklonaler Antikörper und in vitro Funktion [inaugural dissertation]. Ludwig-Maximilians-Universität München; 1994

[22] Gutfeld O, Prus D, Ackerman Z, Dishon S, Linke RP, Levin M, et al. Expression of serum amyloid A, in normal, dysplastic, and neoplastic human colonic mucosa: Implication for a role in colonic tumorigenesis. Journal of Histochemistry and Cytochemistry. 2006;**54**(1):63-73

[23] Urieli-Shoval S, Finci-Yeheskel Z, Eldar I, Linke RP, Levin M, Prus D, et al. Serum amyloid A: Expression throughout human ovarian folliculogenesis and levels in follicular fluid of women undergoing controlled ovarian stimulation. Journal of Clinical Endocrinology and Metabolism. 2013;**98**(12):4970-4978. DOI: 10.1210/jc.2012-1801

[24] Sander LE, Sackett SD, Dierssen U, Beraza N, Linke RP, Müller M, et al. Hepatic acute-phase proteins control innate immune responses during infection by promoting myeloid-derived suppressor cell function. Journal of Experimental Medicine. 2010;**207**(7):1453-1464. DOI: 10.1084/jem.20091474

[25] Linke RP, Meinel A, Chalcroft JP, Urieli-Shoval S. Serum amyloid A (SAA) treatment enhances the recovery of aggravated polymicrobial sepsis in mice, whereas blocking SAA's invariant peptide results in early death. Amyloid. 2017;**24**(suppl 1):149-150

[26] Radelbeck V. Quantifizierung von Serumamyloid-A in einem Mikro-ELISA unter Einsatz monoklonaler Antikörper [dissertation]. Max-Planck-Institution für Biochemie

(Prof. Dr. Robert Huber) und der Medizinischen Fakultät der Ludwigs-Maximilians-Universität München; 1993

[27] Urieli-Shoval S, Linke RP, Matzner Y. Expression and function of serum amyloid A, a major acute-phase protein, in normal and disease states. Current Opinion in Hematology. 2000;**7**(1):64-69 Review

[28] Preciado-Patt L, Levartowsky D, Prass M, Hershkoviz R, Lider O, Fridkin M. Inhibition of cell adhesion to glycoproteins of the extracellular matrix by peptides corresponding to serum amyloid A. Toward understanding the physiological role of an enigmatic protein. European Journal of Biochemistry. 1994;**223**(1):35-42

[29] Gatt ME, Urieli-Shoval S, Preciado-Patt L, Fridkin M, Calco S, Azar Y, et al. Effect of serum amyloid A on selected in vitro functions of isolated human neutrophils. Journal of Laboratory and Clinical Medicine. 1998;**132**(5):414-420

[30] Sackett SD, Otto T, Mohs A, Sander LE, Strauch S, Streetz KL, et al. Myeloid cells require gp130 signaling for protective anti-inflammatory functions during sepsis. FASEB Journal. 2019;**33**(5):6035-6044. DOI: 10.1096/fj.201802118R

[31] Linke RP, Huhn D, Casanova S, Donini U. Immunelectron microscopic identification of human AA-type amyloid: Exploration of various monoclonal AA-antibodies, methods of fixation, embedding and of other parameters for the protein-A gold method. Laboratory Investigation. 1989;**61**:691-697

[32] Urieli-Shoval S, Finci-Yeheskel Z, Dishon S, Galinsky D, Linke RP, Ariel I, et al. Expression of serum amyloid a in human ovarian epithelial tumors: Implication for a role in ovarian tumorigenesis. Journal of Histochemistry and Cytochemistry. 2010;**58**(11):1015-1023. DOI: 10.1369/jhc.2010.956821

[33] Kushner I. The phenomenon of the acute phase response. Annals of the New York Academy of Sciences. 1982;**389**:39-48. Review

[34] Linke RP, Hol PR, Gruys E, Geisel O, Nathrath WB, Trautwein G. Immunohistochemical identification and crossreactions of amyloid-A fibril protein in man and eleven other species. Journal of Comparative Pathology. 1984;**94**(3):339-356

[35] Turnell W, Sarra R, Glover ID, Baum JO, Caspi D, Baltz ML, et al. Secondary structure prediction of human SAA1. Presumptive identification of calcium and lipid binding sites. Molecular Biology & Medicine. 1986;**3**(5):387-407

[36] Uhlar CM, Whitehead AS. Serum amyloid A, the major vertebrate acute-phase reactant. European Journal of Biochemistry. 1999;**265**:501-523

[37] Linke RP. Monoclonal antibodies against amyloid fibril protein AA. Production, specificity, and use for immunohistochemical localization and classification of AA-type amyloidosis. Journal of Histochemistry and Cytochemistry. 1984;**32**(3):322-328

[38] Greunz EM, Lemberger K, Catinaud J, Chenet B, Linke RP, Bräsen JH, et al. Amyloidosis in caracals. Journal of Zoo and Wildlife Medicine. 2020;**51**:202-209

[39] Frankenberger B, Modrow S, Linke RP. Epitope mapping of amyloid-A protein using monoclonal antibodies. In: Natvig JB, Forre O, Husby G, Husebekk A, Skogen B, Sletten K, Westermark P, editors. Amyloid and Amyloidosis. Dordrecht/NL: Kluwer Acad. Publ.; 1991. pp. 87-90

[40] Frankenberger B, Lottspeich F, Linke RP. The monoclonal antibody mc21 recognizes the invariant region of the amyloid-A protein. In: Kisilevsky R, Benson MD, Frangione B, Gaudie J, Muckle TJ, Joung ID, editors. Amyloid and Amyloidosis. New York, London: Parthenon Publishing; 1993. pp. 81-83

[41] Linke RP, Bock V, Valet G, Rothe G. Inhibition of the oxidative burst response of N-formyl peptide-stimulated neutrophils by serum amyloid-A protein. Biochemical and Biophysical Research Communications. 1991;**176**(3):1100-1105

[42] Linke RP, Bock V, Valet G, Rothe G. Increased inhibition of FMLP-induced oxidative burst by serum amyloid-A at 41°C as compared to 37°C. In: Kisilevsky R, Benson MD, Frangione B, Gaudie J, Muckle TJ, Joung ID, editors. New York, London: Parthenon Publishing; 1994. pp. 102-104

[43] Urieli-Shoval S, Shubinsky G, Linke RP, Fridkin M, Tabi I, Matzner Y. Adhesion of human platelets to serum amyloid A. Blood. 2002;**99**(4):1224-1229

[44] Michaeli A, Finci-Yeheskel Z, Dishon S, Linke RP, Levin M, Urieli-Shoval S. Serum amyloid A enhances plasminogen activation: Implication for a role in colon cancer. Biochemical and Biophysical Research Communications. 2008;**368**(2):368-373

[45] Lu J, Yu Y, Zhu I, Cheng Y, Sun PD. Structural mechanism of serum amyloid A-mediated inflammatory amyloidosis. Proceedings of the National Academy of Sciences of the United States of America. 2014;**111**(14):5189-5194. DOI: 10.1073/pnas.1322357111

[46] Köhler G, Milstein C. Continuous cultures of fused cells secreting antibody of predefined specificity. Nature. 1975;**256**(5517):495-497. DOI: 10.1038/256495a0

[47] Frame NM, Gursky O. Structure of serum amyloid A suggests a mechanism for selective lipoprotein binding and functions: SAA as a hub in macromolecular interaction networks. FEBS Letters. 2016;**590**(6):866-879. DOI: 10.1002/1873-3468.12116

[48] Linke RP, Bock V. No change in phagocytosis of normal blood monocytes by serum amyloid A (SAA). In: Kyle RA, Gertz MA, editors. Amyloid and Amyloidosis. New York, London: Parthenon Publ. Group; 1999. pp. 420-422

[49] Reinhard K, Riedemann N. Editorial: Why new approaches that target sepsis need support, p. 3. Text: Fooling a silent killer. European Biotechnology/Autumn Edition. 2016;**15**:15-22

[50] Linke RP. Pharmaceutical composition containing SAA for use in the treatment of acute and chronic dysregulated inflammatory diseases or conditions. In: SAA and Sepsis. Bulletin 2011/39. European Patent Specification. 2011